I DON'T LOOK LIKE WHAT I'VE BEEN THROUGH!

DEBORAH THOMAS, M.DIV

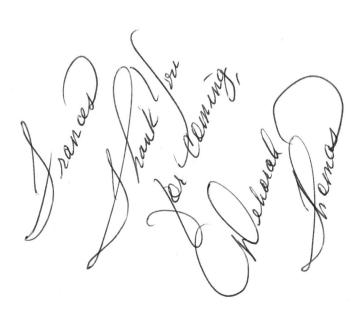

XULON PRESS

Xulon Press
2301 Lucien Way #415
Maitland, FL 32751
407.339.4217
www.xulonpress.com

© 2019 by Deborah Thomas, M.DIV

All rights reserved solely by the author. The author guarantees all contents are original and do not infringe upon the legal rights of any other person or work. No part of this book may be reproduced in any form without the permission of the author. The views expressed in this book are not necessarily those of the publisher.

Scripture quotations taken from:

The King James Version of the Bible (KJV). Public domain.

The Message (MSG). Copyright © 1993, 1994, 1995, 1996, 2000, 2001, 2002 by Eugene H. Peterson.

New English Translation (NET) NET Bible® copyright ©1996-2006 by Biblical Studies Press, L.L.C. http://netbible.com All rights reserved.

Understanding Breast Changes: A Health Guide for Women was originally published by the National Cancer Institute. Public domain.

Printed in the United States of America.

ISBN-13: 978-1-54566-292-2

Table of Contents

Acknowledgements v
Introduction vii
Complacency 1
Excuses 5
Actions 9
Can We Talk? 15
Understanding Breast Changes 33
Bibliography 87
About the Author 89

Acknowledgements

First and foremost, I would like to thank my Lord and Savior for allowing me the opportunity to live and for sustaining me through all my illnesses and hiccups. I would like to thank my children, Marlese, Sean, and Latasha, for their continuing love. Also, I would like to thank my friend and caretaker, Ms. Rita Jenkins, my church family, Advancing the Kingdom Ministries, for your prayers, meals, and words of encouragement, Marquita Outlaw for editing, and Mary Suggs for your unadulterated advice.

Thank you, National Cancer Institute, for allowing me to use your literature. To Sisters Network of Orlando, Inc., you are greatly appreciated for your continuous work in the community for supporting breast cancer victims and survivors.

Last, but not least, my sister Denise for leaving her job and family to take care of me. I appreciate and love you! To all my siblings, nieces and friends thank you, you were all vital to my recovery.

Introduction

While I was sharing my story with several friends of mine, they suggested that I write a book. I was very reluctant, because I realized that my story is not about me, but as the conversation continued, I realized that many of my friends were neglecting their bodies. A clear majority of breast cancer patients stated they kept breast cancer to themselves. I asked the ladies why was it so important that they remain silent? Their responses were "what happens in my house stays there." Through my personal experiences, I realized that I also had learned to suffer in silence because this phrase permeated the household in which I grew up and became the unspoken understanding. This phrase is very dominant in the African-American culture, although many have not realized and I realized that this learned behavior of silence is killing us. The sad thing is that it doesn't matter what situations are presented, whether it's children out of wedlock, some horrific disease, or something as simple as a child getting suspended from school, we were taught to keep silent and keep in the household.

Breast cancer is one of the diseases that no woman wants to hear. In May of 2012, I was diagnosed with breast cancer. Upon hearing the news, my mind went completely blank, and I felt numb. It seemed as if the world had come to a complete stop. I was torn between my desire to hear what I wanted or to accept the reality of what I was told. As I was receiving the disturbing news, the physician and my sister looked at me with this unusual stare, waiting for a response. The only response that I could muster was, "what is the game plan?" Again, I get this unusual stare from my physician. It was as if he was desperately pondering, "how am I going to communicate this, this time to Deborah…as he has many times before, I suspect." With eye's locked with anticipation, we were both waiting on a response from each other. My physician finally broke the silence and asked did I have any other questions and if I had fully understood what he had said. After I was able to get some type of composure, I answered with an adamant yes. This moment was so surreal that my initial reaction was unlike someone who had just been given such detrimental news. I say this, because when I shared the news of my illness; my inner circle of friends' eithers started crying, yelling, gasping and adamantly started denouncing the cancer as it is wasn't what they wanted to hear, and I did neither of those things.

However, before I get any further, I want you to know why it's important to be diligent about our health. We are all formed and transformed by the experiences of our lives. After interviewing women about their health, it became apparent to me that there was a growing disillusionment with how these women treated their bodies. The overall realization that came as a result of these conversations was that women were suffering due to their own silence. Going through this horrific disease (breast cancer) catapulted me into action and an unwavering determination to help other women, especially in the African-American communities, to think differently about their health. I vowed to stop the silence because

Introduction

God allowed me to go through this to help others. This book is written for every breast cancer survivor and for those who are battling this horrific disease. With a biblical perspective, I have included verses to describe how we treat our bodies.

In addition to my own story, I will share stories from other breast cancer survivors—what they did and didn't do. I believe that the compilations of their stories will give a voice and hope to all the women who suffer from this disease. I am a witness that they don't look like what they've been through. If you find you have picked up this book because it has sparked some interest by its title or foreword, trust your instinct that is has something to share for you. If you are familiar with the following phrases or have any of the behaviors listed below, then this book is for you:

- The "C" word should not be discussed….
- Don't speak the word of Cancer and it goes away….
- What happens in this house, stays in this house
- God will take care of it, we don't have to do anything….
- Doctors are not to be trusted….
- Oh, a lump, that's different, it will probably go away….
- Examining my breast for is such a pain….
- Add your excuse or avoidance mechanism to the list…

Then…. get real, get the facts and do everything you can to stay healthy and live a long life. If you're reading this and our stories don't apply to you, I pray that you have the audacity and boldness to share them with someone you know who is neglecting their body, whether they are affected by breast cancer or any other disease. I encourage you to act now. You may be the light that someone is searching for in their dark place.

Chapter 1
Complacency

"The tragedy of life is not found in failure but complacency. Not in you doing too much, but doing too little. Not in you living above your means, but below your capacity. It's not failure but aiming too low, that is life's greatest tragedy."   –Benjamin E. Mays

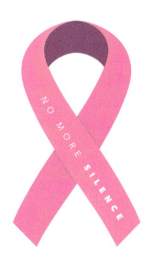

> ***After this there was a feast of the Jews; and Jesus went up to Jerusalem.² Now there is at Jerusalem by the sheep market a pool, which is called in the Hebrew tongue Bethesda, having five porches.³ In these lay a great multitude of impotent folk, of blind, halt, withered, waiting for the moving of the water.⁴ For an angel went down at a certain season into the pool, and troubled the water: whosoever then first after the troubling the water stepped in was made whole of whatsoever disease he had.⁵ And a certain man was there, which had an infirmity thirty and eight years. John 5:1-5 King James Version (KJV)***

When examining this scripture, I compare this to how we treat our bodies. So many women live while receiving constant warning signs from their bodies yet will not take the initiative to change their situations. In hopes that their symptoms will go away, they are conditioned to a life of security, conformity, and complacency, putting off wellness checks, believing that nothing appears to be wrong and despite common misconception, nothing is more dangerous than neglecting the body. We become very complacent about our health, especially women. It is a well-known fact that we, as women, put everyone before ourselves. It's insane how we can put our needs and wants behind those of others. If you are a wife or a mother, you are continually making sacrifices for the people around you, without realizing that you are losing yourself amongst the chaos.

Look at this scripture closely. The man with an infirmity went to Jerusalem the same time every year because he knew that the waters would be stirred. It is believed in that region than an angel would come a certain time every year and rouse the water. Whoever stepped in first got healed. Can you imagine a mob scene where hundreds of people are trying to get into the pool and here lies a man with a debilitating illness trying to get in? This man had been doing this for thirty-eight years hoping to get assistance from someone. I can only imagine the frustration he encountered. Thirty-eight years is a long time to be nursing a disease and waiting to be cured. He never saw any changes, but he could always be expected to get into the water. His state of complacency is a prime example of insanity. Albert Einstein is broadly credited with exclaiming, "The definition of insanity is doing the same thing over and again but expecting different results."[1] Here, we see a man waiting and hoping for numerous years, and as he waits and his life becomes stagnant.

Unfortunately, this is how we treat our bodies. No one knows our bodies better than ourselves. We know something is wrong, but we become stagnant, ignoring the signs and waiting and hoping that illnesses or pains will go away. We need to be diligent and pay attention to the new pain, sensations, abnormality of skin discolorations, lumps in breasts, extreme fatigue and headaches, just to name a few. We become so complacent that we are unable to see the warning signs our bodies are displaying. Our lives become the sentence, "As soon as I…then I will do…" We can fill in the blanks. I don't know about you, but if I knew that the waters were troubled the same time every year, I would step into the water a day earlier, even if I had to look like a prune. As women, we do the same thing. We know that we should get our wellness checks every year; however, we continue

---

[1] http://wisdomquotes.com/albert-einstein-qoutes

to put it off for so many other reasons. Women, if you have problems remembering, I implore you to make an appointment on a significant date (i.e. your birth month or anniversary month). Examine yourself and what have you been complacent about, especially your health. I once heard a man say, "There is no such thing as complacency"; he said it means that you purposed in your heart that your goals or plans are not important enough. Wow, what a profound statement. I started applying this idea to plans that I had been putting off such as writing this book and retirement. I asked myself, "Is it important enough?" If it wasn't, I started prioritizing them from the most important to the least, and it was amazing how much I could get done after I purposed in my heart to just start. Had I not purposed to get an examination every year, I would have been one of the statistics, finding out that I had breast cancer too late to give myself a fighting chance for survival. Thank God for wisdom! Ladies, it's time we take responsibility for our lives, because no one else will.

Chapter 2

Excuses

"Not managing your health and making excuses are two bad habits that leads to destruction." —Deborah Thomas, M.DIV

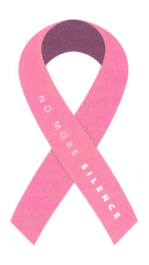

> **When Jesus saw him lie and knew that he had been now a long time in that case, he saith unto him, Wilt thou be made whole?[7] The impotent man answered him, Sir, I have no man, when the water is troubled, to put me into the pool: but while I am coming, another steppeth down before me. John 5:6-7, KJV**

In this passage, Jesus asked the man if he wanted to be made whole. The man replied that he was waiting on a man. **What an excuse!** This man had the capability to get to the pool for thirty-eight years, but he was waiting on a man to put him in. My question is how did he get to the pool? How many excuses do we use for not going to the doctor? The dictionary definition of "excuse" is "to make allowance for a shortcoming; to overlook; to serve as justification for; to vindicate."[2]

This spirit of excuses is nothing new under the sun. As we look at Adam and Eve in Genesis 3:12-13, we read that they each came up with excuses for why they were disobedient. "The man said, 'The woman you put here with me—she gave me some fruit from the tree, and I ate it.' Then the LORD God said to the woman, 'What is this you have done?' The woman said, 'The serpent deceived me, and I ate.'" As we deny or and make excuses for our negligence of our health, we are unable to formulate a plan to move forward. Making excuses will not make our illness or pain go away. Excuses seem like valid reasons not to do something, but perhaps you should take a closer look before you decide to make one up. Excuses are negative thoughts derived from fear. If your negative thoughts go unchallenged, you are giving them

---

[2] Webster Dictionary (definition of excuse, 1828)

power; then because you have accepted them, the subtleness becomes your truth. Negativity creates indecisiveness, which results in complacency. The definition of complacency is self-satisfaction especially when accompanied by unawareness of actual dangers or deficiencies.[3] Being consistent and diligent about your health doesn't just happen. We must take the necessary steps that include being diligent and decisive, planning and setting aside time to execute the plan. The sad thing about this truth is that millions of people use excuses every day.

Fear paralyzes your thoughts and actions. Fear is based on your perception of what the outcome will be. The truth of the matter is that we don't know what the next second will bring. In the book of Exodus, Moses gave many excuses for why he couldn't lead the Israelites out of Egypt.

> Moses said to the Lord, "Lord, I am not a man of words. I have never been. Even now since You spoke to Your servant, I still am not. For I am slow in talking and it is difficult for me to speak." Then the Lord said to him, "Who has made man's mouth? Who makes a man not able to speak or hear? Who makes one blind or able to see? Is it not I, the Lord? So, go now. And I will be with your mouth. I will teach you what to say." But Moses said, "O Lord, I ask of You, send some other person."[4]

The guaranteed result of making excuses is the inability to act appropriately. God wants us to move from fear to faith.

---

[3] Webster Dictionary (definition of complacency, 1828)
[4] Exodus 4:10-14 New Living Translation

That means that actions are significant if it is our desire to have a different outcome. Don't allow your excuses to keep you from reaching your healthy you.

Chapter 3

Actions

*"Your beliefs become your thoughts,
Your thoughts become your words,
Your words become your actions,
Your actions become your habits,
Your habits become your values,
Your values become your destiny."*
—Mahatma Gandhi

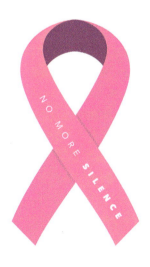

> ***Jesus saith unto him, Rise, take up thy bed, and walk. And immediately the man was made whole, and took up his bed, and walked: and on the same day was the sabbath. John 5:8-9 KJV***

According to Webster's Dictionary, action is defined as "something done or perform or an act that one consciously wills; and that may be characterized by physical or mental activity."[5] In this scripture, we see a man who decided to make a choice and act on it. Believe that we develop this mentality by rehearsing in our minds that we're going to do something about our health. We practice conversations in our mind, such as "I'll go when I get some money, or maybe the symptoms will go away or even say we're going to see a doctor" until that becomes just a saying. We often used the coined statement, "Actions speaks louder than words." How is it that this just becomes a cliché in our life? Remember, our words become our actions. What you do is more important than what you say. Action requires us to purposely pursue something. James says it so eloquently,

> ***[Faith in Action] Dear friends, do you think you'll get anywhere in this if you learn all the right words but never do anything? Does merely talking about faith indicate that a person really has it? For instance, you come upon an old friend dressed in rags and half-starved and say, "Good morning, friend! Be clothed in Christ! Be filled with the Holy Spirit!" and walk off***

---

[5] Webster Dictionary (definition of action, 1828)

> **without providing so much as a coat or a cup of soup—where does that get you? Isn't it obvious that God-talk without God-acts is outrageous nonsense?**[6]

Chapter three, "***Taking Action***" of my book, is probably one of the most important chapters in this book. I am calling all readers to action by developing a health practice that could lead to a productive and healthy life. The problem with action is that it gets distorted in the busyness of our lives. We have become so accustomed to our busyness that we have trained our ears and bodies not to listen the warnings of pain until it's too late. Listening is a discipline that must be acquired to live. Most people equate listening with love and respect. It is imperative that we stop being silent and start listening. Despite all the awareness and prevention walks, conventions, publications, concerts, etc., we continue to ignore the warning signs (pain, unusual lumps, etc.) that our bodies are displaying and do business as usual. Steps that we can take is forming a community amongst our peers, to hold each other accountable. If you have gone through various health issues, there are a lot of support systems out there to assist. I belong to Sisters Network® Inc. of Orlando. Becoming a member was one of the best things that I could have done. This organization is committed to increasing local and national attention to the devastating impact that breast cancer has in the African American community.

> This organization was founded by Karen Eubanks Jackson, Founder/CEO of Sisters Network® Inc. (SNI) is recognized nationally as

---

[6] James 2:14-26, The Message Bible

a true visionary, leader in the African American breast cancer movement and a 23-year breast cancer survivor. Sisters Network is the nation's only African American breast cancer survivorship organization. Jackson continues to lead Sisters Network's nationwide effort to focus the spotlight on increasing breast cancer awareness in the African American community. The organization provides standardized national educational outreach programs; survivor & family support; empowerment; hope and financial assistance to thousands of women annually through its national network of survivor-run affiliate chapters located in 22 states.[7]

Sister's Network was vital to my continuing survival. I was able to form relationships with women, who not only look like me, but who also understood the African-American culture. During the meetings, discussions took place about how there are disparities of medical treatments that exist between different ethnic groups, whereas in the African-American culture there is such a huge difference in how we are treated physically and the financial support that we receive. I am a woman who is perceived to be very strong in nature. My friends always say, you are such a strong woman. They only saw the outer appearance. My friends and colleagues were unaware of my insecurities, my fears and my struggle to maintain hope while battling breast cancer. SNI was an outlet for me to express my fears and to gain strength, support and hope. Participating with this organization allowed me to be vulnerable without the fear of criticism. There is so much

---

[7] http://www.sistersnetworkinc.org/founder.html

positivity and trustworthiness with the women in my group who are walking or have walked through the triumphs as well as the struggles; that makes the fight with breast cancer a little bit easier to deal with. Not only did they provide the support needed, it also taught me how important it is to give back to the community. I was able to host a health fair at my church and provide fifteen women with free mammograms. I realized through this struggle that it wasn't about me but all about God. He allowed me to go through this, so I can be a living testimony to how great He is.

Through my processes and speaking with other survivors, I realized that not only do we proactively examine our health issues, but that there were women who have gone through traumatic health issues and did not have a recovery plan. This is also part of the action plan. We need to first accept the situation for what it is and determine if we want to live. This is vital to how we determine our action plan. Exercise, eat a balanced diet, maintain a healthy weight, get good sleep, reduce stress, avoid tobacco and limit the amount of alcohol you drink. For cancer survivors, some healthy behaviors may lower the risk of recurrence and improve survival.[8] Make it simple and put it on paper! This gives you specific and measurable goals. Even if we hit a rough spot in our recovery, having a visual plan laid out gives us a push to get back up and try to obtain the goals that were developed, thus becoming our road map to reach our destination. You must set a reasonable time frame to reach these goals. Make sure your plan consists of all the pertinent information that is needed—for example, your doctor appointments, your support group with names and numbers, your medication dosage, your insurance information, and a change of healthy living—and please give a

---

[8] www.cancer.org/healthy

copy of your plan to your accountability partner. Review and measure your progress daily. You can revise your plan as needed. Remember to celebrate when you obtain one of your desired goals. Finally, share the information. Attached at the end of this book is a wealth of information that was provided by the National Cancer Institute. The attachment provides information on understanding the anatomy of the breast and a health guide to help you through the process.

As I stated earlier, one of our communities' biggest woes is silence. **LISTEN** and **SILENT** have the same letters; choose which combination of these you will use. ***"But do you want to know, O foolish man, that faith without works is dead?"***[9] This passage is stating that the lack of action is revealing unchanged habits. We can't expect different results when we do the same thing. This is called insanity. Over the last six years and during my time interviewing women who have had breast cancer or some other illness, I have learned that these women knew something was wrong but thought that their problem would just go away in time. These ladies became so complacent and willingly put themselves in a state of denial. I always say, "Denial is not the river (The Nile River)." Ladies and gentlemen, please get your wellness checks; it's a form of action. "It may not be in your power, may not be in your time, that there'll be any fruit. But that doesn't mean you stop doing the right thing. You may never know what results come from your **action**. But if you do nothing, there will be no result."[10] In the above-mentioned scripture, Jesus commanded the man to action. As the man responded, he became cured. All sicknesses are not unto death; however, if left unnoticed or if no action is taken, death could very well be the result.

---

[9] James 2:20
[10] http://www.goodreadquotes.com/mahatmagandhi

Chapter 4

Can We Talk?

"You know that you've healed an issue when you can talk about it and you're not weeping, when you can speak to it and identify the lesson. You know that you've healed an issue when, having gone through that, has a benefit that you live today.

—Iyanla Vanzant

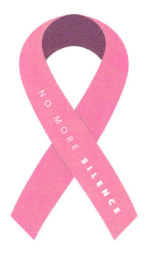

> **"And they overcame him by the blood of the Lamb and by the word of their testimony, and they did not love their lives to the death." Revelations 12:11, KJV**

Life stories do not simply give a cure to one's illness; however, by telling these stories, my prayer is that they give someone hope and encourage others to manage their health. In this chapter, we have women who have survived breast cancer and are willing to share their experiences.

Emma Davis, Survivor Story -

In April 1989, doctors told me I had a negative mammogram. Four months later, at the age of forty-four, I found a lump in my right breast. To my surprise, the diagnosis was Stage One DCIS breast cancer. Immediately, my emotional door flew open…tears, shock, and disbelief. I thought to myself, *Maybe the test results were meant for someone else*. How could I have breast cancer when there was no family history of any kind of this cancer? My treatment plan consisted of a right mastectomy and four months of chemotherapy. I experienced the common side effects of chemotherapy. Seeing my hair on my pillow and falling out as I combed it was pretty upsetting to me. Suffering through severe bouts of nausea and dehydration was also a tough time during my treatment period. I soon realized my lifestyle had to change because the enemy (cancer) wanted to take my livelihood. From the day of my diagnoses, I took advantage of the scripture "Pray without ceasing" (1 Thess. 5:17). With my faith in God and support from my awesome husband, children, church family, and friends, I was on course to defeat the enemy…so I thought.

Fast forward to August 2000. I felt a lump in my right chest wall where I previously had the mastectomy. The medical report confirmed my worst fear: cancer had returned…Stage Four diagnosis. This time, I was emotionally, mentally, and spiritually stronger after receiving the news. I focused on the positive things in my life, like continuing to work in the Lord's church, seeing my grandchildren grow up and marry, and giving back to the community. My doctors treated the cancer more aggressively by giving me six months of weekly chemotherapy and six weeks of radiation treatments. The fear of dealing with severe nausea again troubled my spirit. However, I prayed earnestly to God and remembered His Word: "God has not given us a spirit of fear, but of power and of love and of a sound mind" (2 Tim. 1:7). My treatment phase was less painful this time. About one year prior to my reoccurrence of breast cancer, I lost my main supporter, my husband. As always, my two wonderful children, Herman (Slim) and April, along with other family members, rallied around me as I began to fight this enemy again.

I have been cancer free now for fourteen years. Praise God! My journey with breast cancer didn't end when the treatment ended. I made several life-changing decisions for the better. I retired from Lockheed Martin in 2002. I have a new appreciation for life and a passion for helping others. A typical week in my life consists of providing coats for inner-city kids, volunteering at University of Florida Cancer Center Orlando Health, and cooking meals for Fresh Start homeless shelter. I am also a member of the Orlando Chapter of Sisters Network Inc. This is a survivorship organization committed to bringing breast health awareness to the African American community.

I now recognize that some challenges along my journey were truly blessings. I am eternally grateful to God, who is true to His promises. I give a shout out to my medical team at UF Health Cancer Center for the successful treatment plan to attack "the enemy." I also appreciate the compassionate care of their medical staff I received as a patient. Most of all, I am indebted to my family and friends for their prayers and support. Now I am joyfully surviving and thriving in remission today. **Praise the Lord!**

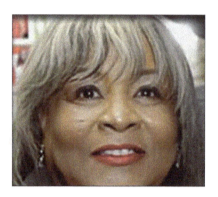

Loretta Broome Moore, Survivor Story

I'm Loretta Broome Moore, and this is my story:

In March 2005, while visiting my son and his family in Missouri, while playing with my grandson, he butted his head against my breast; that is when I noticed the lump. My vacation was shot, just thinking of the worst.

After having several tests, my worst fear came to reality. I was diagnosed with DCIS Stage Two in my right breast. I thought the world was coming to an end. I just couldn't believe this was happening to someone who had yearly physicals and did monthly breast exams. I had just gone through this with my husband, who was diagnosed in 2002 and lost his battle in 2003. I began to question God, and then I remembered Romans 8:28: *"And we know that all things work together for the good to them that love GOD, to*

them that are called according to his purpose." And my purpose was to beat this deadly disease, so I could do ministry and help others. My support team was great: medical, family, co-workers, church family, and friends supported me through it all. I opted to have a mastectomy and have been in remission for thirteen years. I was given a special gift during my treatment—Jazz, my dog, and she was great therapy for me. God's grace and mercy have brought me through every obstacle of this journey. I am presently involved in Orlando's Chapter of Sisters Network Inc., an Africa-American survivorship organization. Our mission is to "Stop the Silence."

Catherine Polk, Survivor Story

My name is Catherine Polk. It was October 3, 2017 when I received the news that I had breast cancer. I had no symptoms. I noticed fatty tissue under my left arm as I bathed. I said, "This is probably like the fatty tissue that was on my back in 1998," and since it was near my breast, I thought that I should get it checked out anyway. I prayed about it and went to the doctor.

I did not think too much about it; I had some fatty tissue on my back in 1998, all benign, and kept checking to see if it was growing. I decided to speak to my doctor about it, and my husband was with me; it was on from there. The doctor sent me for a mammogram, then a Cat-Scan and Muga-Scan, then a biopsy. Test results showed a diagnosis as cancer.

My initial feelings were disgust and disappointment. I began to think about those that I have known that had cancer, and knowing what had happened to them, I began to talk to the children about it and really felt just a bit out of it. I did not believe that it could be cancer, yet I was feeling fine. I realized, after taking into further consideration that you do not have to feel like there is anything wrong, that all those test results were telling me something.

I elected to receive chemotherapy. I had three high doses of chemotherapy. This treatment seemed to just about kill me. I lost thirty pounds in a three-month period. My body could not function, I ached all over, my bones became very weak, I could not eat very much of anything, and I began to get nausea at the smell of food and coffee and could not partake in very much. I begin to pray and ask God for help, to lead me as to what I was to do. I know that He is a healer, and I do not believe He would have me to continue to allow my body to be abused the way it was. I began to feel like I was being tortured. I prayed for God to enable me to stop the treatments, and I asked God to heal me, for I knew that He could do it as He has done so many times before. The Lord assured me that He can cure cancer. I just needed to walk in faith and not doubt or be afraid. I was convinced that it was just a test. We talk about how much we trust God, yet we allow ourselves to put so much trust in man. I was praying and trusting God even more. The last test result was that the cancer had shrunk, and they wanted to do surgery and radiation; however, God has healed me, and I am walking in that assurance.

I was asked the question, "Now that you have survived, what are your feelings?" Now, I feel fine. Trusting God for life and not death, I shall live until He says, "Come on home, my child." I am keeping the faith, and eating properly, trying to rest more in Him, and being led by His Spirit and nothing else.

The other question was, "What advice would you give to women today?" Make sure you take time to take care of yourself. Do keep check on your body, and don't be afraid; there is simply nothing too hard for God. He is Yahweh Rapha. Let His peace abides in your hearts.

Love One Another! "Let the peace of God rule in your hearts."

Pray ACTS: A–Adoration C–Confession T–Thanksgiving S–Supplication

Melanie Mack, Survivor Story

When I turned forty, I committed to checking my breasts on my birth date of each month so that I would not forget. This gave me a baseline understanding about what my breasts felt like normally. So, when a lump showed up four years later, I knew right away that something was wrong. I shared it with my doctor, who was able to confirm the lump that I found. He said that it was not the size or shape that he would expect if it were cancerous, however, he wanted me to come back in another six months to see if it had changed in any way. It had changed a little, so he wanted me to have a biopsy. I scheduled the appointment, then cancelled it a week prior to the procedure because I was too busy at work, it was the holidays, and I had too much going on. In short, I was afraid.

That's when my husband, my sister, and my manager started pushing me to re-schedule. They argued with me, took away my excuses, and made me feel like it was life or death...and it was. It took me another three or four months to re-schedule that appointment and the results came back inconclusive. My doctor explained that inconclusive is not an answer, so he wanted me to have a second biopsy. He had to fight for me because my insurance carrier would not approve another one, and he was relentless! I had the second biopsy in June 2013, and on July 31, 2013 the surgeon started our conversation with, "Mrs. Mack I am so sorry to have to tell you this, but the results of your biopsy are back, and you've been diagnosed with breast cancer."

I learned that I had two different kinds of breast cancers in my left breast—one that was estrogen-based and slow growing, but the other was much more aggressive. The original lump that I found was benign. The cancers were found in the surrounding tissue, so had I not found the benign lump, I may not have been diagnosed with Stage One breast cancer. We found it early!

Ultimately, I had a double mastectomy, breast tissue expanders for a year, twenty-one weeks of chemotherapy, an Oophorectomy to remove my ovaries (due to the estrogen-based cancer), Diep flap breast reconstruction, and a host of other treatments and procedures over the past five years. Yes, this is my fifth anniversary as a breast cancer survivor! By the grace of God, and the love and support of my husband, children, family and close friends, sorority sisters, and Sisters Network.

Sisters Network, Inc. is an organization that brings attention to the deadly impact that breast cancer is having on the Black community. These women embraced me and let me know that I was not alone. According to www.breastcancer.org, "In women under 45, breast cancer is more common in African-American women than white women. Overall, African-American women are more likely to die of breast cancer."

Breast cancer is deadly, but it does not necessarily mean a death sentence. Women must love ourselves enough to become more familiar with our breasts than our doctors and partners. Of all the roles that I play—wife, mother, sister, daughter, friend, colleague—none is more important than the one I was born with...myself. I am important. I am a survivor! And so are you.

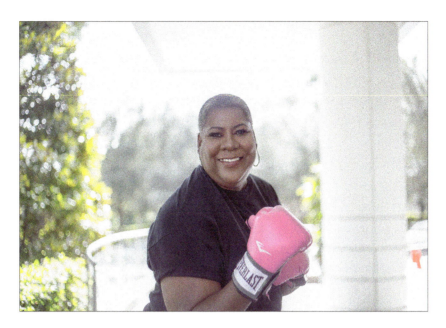

My name is Deborah Thomas, and I am the author of this book. I'm very reserved and am known for having a calm nature. I very seldom lose my temper and am an introvert. I am a woman of strong faith. There are times when this faith gets shaken to the core. When this happens, I have learned to rely on one of my favorite scriptures: ***"Be strong and of good courage, do not fear nor be afraid of them; for the Lord your God, He is the One who goes with you. He will not leave you nor forsake you" (Deut. 31:6).***

Through the various trials and struggles with this horrific disease, I was catapulted to write this book because of the stories and experiences I encountered. In May 2012, I had my wellness check. This is something I've been doing for a long time since my mother died of pancreatic cancer. I often wondered if she ever had any signs. I can't recall my mother ever going to the doctor or even being sick. If she was, she too suffered in silence. By the time she discovered that she had cancer, it was too late. The oncologist told the family that she had about six months to live. She lasted twenty days. Even though it is said that pancreatic cancer is hard to detect, I often pondered if she had gone to get wellness checks every year, would they have found it earlier? I then vowed, that I would get wellness checks every year. Part of my wellness check was to have a mammogram. However, we still must be diligent about our health, and if you have a history of breast cancer or any other genetic disease, sometimes things need to go further. Here are some known facts about breast mammography:

A negative x-ray report should not delay if a dominant or clinically suspicious mass is present. 4-8 percent of cancers are not identified by x-ray.

- A negative report may reinforce clinical impression.
- Adenosis and dense breast may obscure an underlying neoplasm.
- False positive results average 6-10 percent.
- It is the **responsibility** of the **patient** to supply the location and date of last screening mammography procedure.
- Mammography is important in sustaining ongoing health.

My gynecologist called me and stated there was a significant change in my breast from the previous year. He sent me out for an ultrasound of the area, and a mass was found, and calcification was present in both breasts. Immediately, he recommended that I get further testing. Having done all the tests, the result was that the mass was benign. Excited about the news, I shared my experiences with my inner circle. However, my doctor called me back in and stated that there was a mass and he should just remove it. His words were,

"We don't need anything growing in your body that doesn't belong there." So, I had a lumpectomy done. I was very ignorant to the process, so I thought that after it was removed, all would be well. Remember the six points that I mentioned in the above paragraph? I had no symptoms before the wellness check that would have even indicated that I had breast cancer.

After the removal of the mass, I went in to visit the doctor for a follow-up of the procedure, thinking he was going to check the incision and make sure no infection was present. My sister and best friend drove me to the doctor's appointment. They indicated they would be in the waiting room until I finished my follow-up appointment. After the doctor came in and as I was getting prepared, my sister barged into the room. She startled both of us, because we weren't expecting someone else to come into the room. My immediate response was, "What are you doing?" If anyone knows my sister, they know that she can be very loud and rumbustious. She responded, "I need to know!" I told her that I'm an adult and not her child. However, through various word changes, I elected to allow her to stay because the poor doctor didn't know what to do or say. After the commotion settled down, the doctor later went on to say that the mass was hiding the cancer. Here again, my sister barged in and stated, "The devil is a liar." I was still sitting there, trying to grasp what he had just said. So, when I was able to get a word in, I asked what his proposed solution and plan was for attacking this disease. After regaining his composure because of the earlier commotion and my initial lack or response The doctor immediately started giving me my options and all the specifications of the stage I was in. **Thank God!** I was diagnosed with Ductal carcinoma in situ (DCIS) of the left breast, which is the lowest stage of breast cancer. It is non-invasive but if left untreated can eventually become invasive and problematic.

At this point, I was glad my sister came in, because in that moment, everything was surreal. She immediately started asking detailed questions about the disease. Still being defiant, she was adamant that based on her faith, what the doctor stated was lie. About a few days later, I had the opportunity to digest all that was said, and then the light bulb went on. How did she know to ask those detailed questions? I began to interrogate her about her knowledge of this disease. She went on to tell me that she had battled breast cancer about a year ago. I was livid because she didn't think it was important for me to know. Remember, I stated earlier, "Whatever goes on in my house stays there." This detrimental phrase has caused dysfunctional behavior that had the potential to be harmful and even deadly to me if I hadn't been diligent about my health.

I was later referred to an oncologist. His recommendation was to have ten to twelve weeks of radiation and chemotherapy or have a bilateral mastectomy. He then referred me out to a radiation oncologist. I made an appointment. My husband at the time and I went in for the consultation. As we were seated, the doctor asked me why I was there. A little taken back by her question, I asked, "What do you mean by that?" She knew I was referred from one of her colleagues. I answered that the oncologist sent me to her. She then made the remark, "That's very textbook." After about an hour of consultation, I was still not quite sure what decision to make. During this consultation, she told me there was an 80 to 85 percent chance that she could get it all; however, if she could not, I would have to have a mastectomy. So, at the end of the consultation, my husband asked her, "If this was your plight, what would you recommend?" She stated that because of the location and the odds, she would opt to have the mastectomy. After much prayer, I decided to have a double mastectomy.

After making the decision to have surgery, I elected to share the news with some of my praying friends. I was later told by some of them that they were afraid, some cried, and some didn't know what to do. Their best friend could be dying, and it was out of their control. I want you to know, there was some fear, but God didn't give me a sense that I was dying. It never really crossed my mind. However, I have a friend name Pam who came to my house to pray before surgery. In that room were my daughter Marlese, Rita, and myself. Pam prayed for each of them and gave them a Word from the Lord. I'm looking at her thinking, *what did the Lord say about me and when are you going to pray for me? I'm the one who is sick.* She never prayed, however, she turned to me and said, "This didn't catch the Lord by surprise." Along with my favorite scripture, I held on to that phrase, and even now when anything goes on in my life, I continue to stand on that scripture and phrase.

After the surgery, I was told that the approximate healing would take six to eight weeks. I had the surgery in July and returned home in about three days. On the third day and after several visitations, I became very cold. My daughter LaTasha came home, and I instructed her to get me some blankets. She became very concerned because I'm never cold. She walked up to the bed to cover me and realized that my body was emitting heat. She then went to the discharge information and began to read it. She returned to me and asked if I had a thermometer. My response was, "I haven't seen a thermometer since you were a tot." She immediately went to the local store and purchase one. My temperature was well over 103 degrees.

She got me up and went around the corner to get help and rushed me back to the hospital. I later found out that I had Sepsis, and it was in the bloodstream. Numerous doctors and nurses were rushing in, trying to find the antibiotics that could attack this infection before it killed me. During the mastectomy, I was told that they took a lymph node out of my left arm to have it examined because it was swollen, and they needed to figure out the extent of cancer involvement. Cancer in the lymph nodes is associated with an increased risk of having cancer cells in other parts of your body. Because of this procedure, I was told that I could not have blood pressure, IVs, or any type of procedure to the left arm for a period of ten years. Because of the numerous times they had placed IVs and taken blood in the right arm, my veins began to collapse. On the fourth day of my hospital visit, the nurses and doctors finally were able to find a vein and the right medication to subdue the infection. Thank God for another miracle. Remember, earlier I said this would take six to eight weeks, but the process became longer.

After getting out of the hospital, my doctor told me that they had to wait six to eight months before they could start the reconstruction process. They said that they had to make sure my body was completely healed, and that no infections. were present. I couldn't go back to work because of the potential risk of getting sick from other germs and having a relapse. At this point, I became very frustrated because I'm usually a very busy person, and I couldn't sit home and do nothing. It became so bad that I started reading textbooks from college, painting by number, and even putting together jigsaw puzzles. I did anything constructive to occupy my time and to prevent my mind from wandering into dark places.

After about six months, I returned to the reconstruction surgeon, and he performed surgery to put the expanders in.

This process is done to expand the breast skin and muscle to the desired size of the breast. Once the process is completed, surgery to put in the permanent implants is usually performed four to six weeks later. However, this didn't happen in the time frame that I had expected. About three weeks into the expansion process, I awoke in the middle of the night and realized that my shirt was wet. I didn't get alarmed because I had an appointment the following day. I went to the plastic surgeon's office and explained what had happened. The nurse examined the breast and realized the stitched area was opening. She made the decision not to expand and to wait a few days, and she would let the doctor know. I left the office expecting to return on Friday to continue the expansion process.

I went home that day and took a nap. At about 4:30 in the afternoon, my phone rang. I looked at the caller ID and realized it was the plastic surgeon's office whom I saw earlier that day. I ignored the call thinking it was a reminder of my upcoming appointment. I went back to sleep, and the Holy Spirit woke me up at 4:55 p.m. and told me to check my messages. I immediately checked and heard a message stating that plans had changed and that I needed to call the office immediately. I called, got the answering service, and was patched through. I was told at that moment that I had to be in surgery at 5:30 a.m. the next day. At that point, I was given no other information.

I called my oldest daughter, Marlese, and told her of the situation. She took me to the hospital, and I told her that I wanted to know what was going on before I was sedated. The doctor came in and explained that because of my history with infections, he wanted to go in and clean around the area to make sure there were no infections present. He then assured me that if there were no complications, I would be done by 7:30 a.m. and back home by noon. I went through the surgery, and when I awoke, the first thing I did was thank God, and then I looked at the clock. I turned to my daughter and said, "He was right; it's 7:30." She laughed and said, "It's 7:30 *p.m.*" I was surprised and asked her what had happened. She informed me that when they went in, the expanders had exploded, and infections were present, but everything was okay; however, the process needed to stop for another six months. Remember, this was supposed to be a six-to-eight-week process. I was frustrated and thankful at the same time.

As I was going through this, my job was in jeopardy. I had exhausted all my sick leave, vacation time, and Family Medical Leave Act (FMLA). This is a labor law requiring covered employers to provide employees with job protection and unpaid leave for qualified medical and family reasons. I begged my doctor to let me go back to work, and reluctantly, he allowed me to work part-time. This didn't sit well with my employer, and I was told that if I couldn't give them a specific date to return to work, I should resign, or the employer would terminate me. After being at a job for over fifteen years, you would think that loyalty would come into play. However, God always has a ram in the bush. The company had just hired a new director who happened to be over my department. I went to see her and explained my situation. Up until I was diagnosed with breast cancer, I was always at work and had worked in several departments when I was needed. She later said that she would examine my work history and decide on a solution. She then told me to get well and not worry about the job. God is awesome.

The time finally came for me to get the implants, and I'm grateful that all went well. Through these numerous surgeries and painful processes, I am truly grateful to the Almighty God that I don't look like what I've been through. Although

I interviewed several ladies who have survived, some were not ready to share their stories. Some felt guilty for ignoring their bodies until it was almost too late, and some still suffered from the syndrome of keeping things silent. Through the compilations of these testimonies, I hope you are compelled to get your wellness checks.

The next pages provides a wealth of information from the National Cancer Institute, which allowed me to reproduce their pamphlet in case you or someone you know needs any help. Be blessed and take care of your bodies. Please **listen** to them and don't be **silent**. Remember, both words have the same letters.-

Understanding Breast Changes

A Health Guide for Women

National Cancer Institute

I Don't Look Like What I've Been Through!

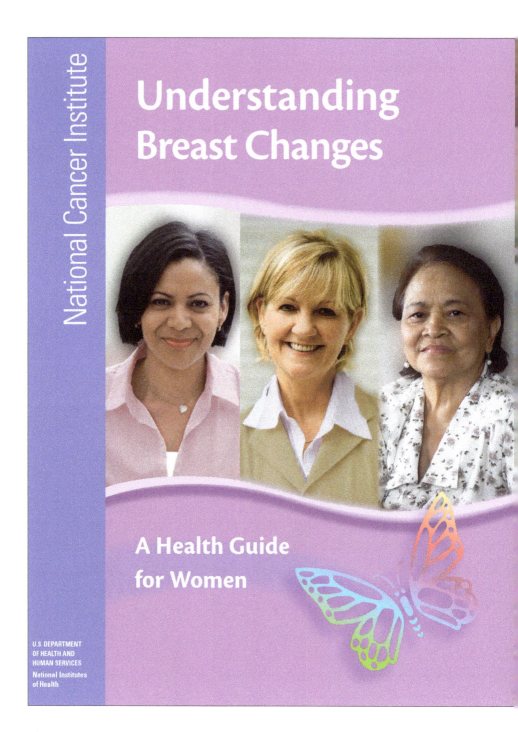

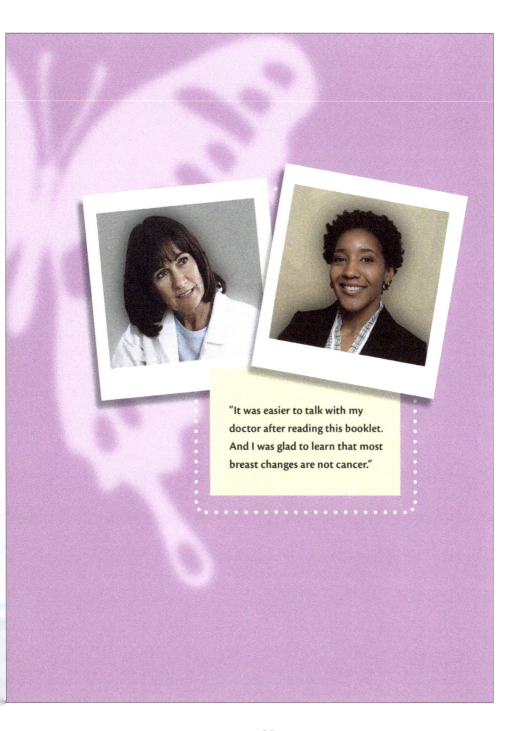

"It was easier to talk with my doctor after reading this booklet. And I was glad to learn that most breast changes are not cancer."

I Don't Look Like What I've Been Through!

Table of Contents

Introduction 1

Anatomy of the breast 2

Chapters

1. Breast and lymphatic system basics 3

2. Check with your health care provider
about breast changes 4

3. Breast changes during your lifetime that
are not cancer 7

4. Finding breast changes 9

5. Getting your mammogram results 13

6. Follow-up tests to diagnose breast changes 16

7. Breast changes and conditions:
Getting follow-up test results 20

8. Getting the support you need 24

Breast conditions and follow-up care 25

Resources to learn more 29

Words to know 31

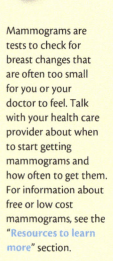

Mammograms are tests to check for breast changes that are often too small for you or your doctor to feel. Talk with your health care provider about when to start getting mammograms and how often to get them. For information about free or low cost mammograms, see the "Resources to learn more" section.

Words To Know

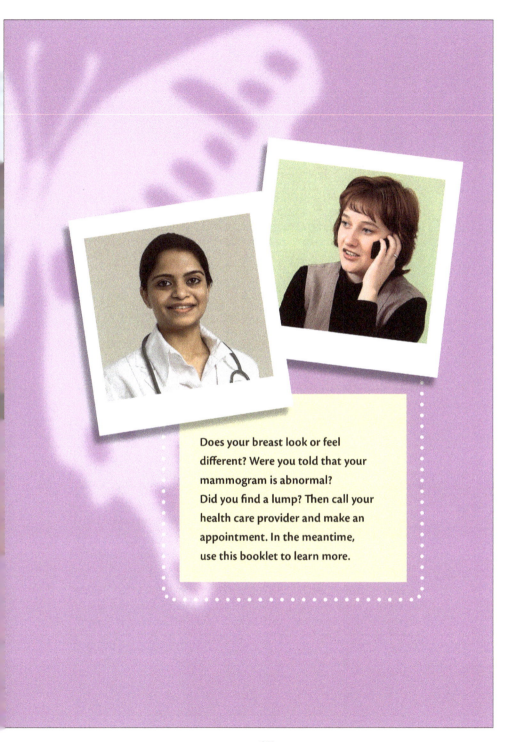

Does your breast look or feel different? Were you told that your mammogram is abnormal? Did you find a lump? Then call your health care provider and make an appointment. In the meantime, use this booklet to learn more.

Introduction

You may be reading this booklet because you, or your health care provider, found a **breast** lump or other breast change. Keep in mind that breast changes are very common. Most breast changes are not **cancer**. But it is very important to get the follow-up tests that your health care provider asks you to.

What are breast changes?

Many breast changes are changes in how your breast or **nipple** looks or feels. You may notice a lump or firmness in your breast or under your arm. Or perhaps the size or shape of your breast has changed. Your nipple may be pointing or facing inward (inverted) or feeling tender. The skin on your breast, **areola**, or nipple may be scaly, red, or swollen. You may have **nipple discharge**, which is an **abnormal** fluid coming from the nipple.

If you have these or other breast changes, talk with your health care provider to get these changes checked as soon as possible.

This booklet can help you take these steps:

- Call your health care provider to make an appointment as soon as you notice any breast changes.
- Go back to see your health care provider if your **mammogram** result is abnormal.
- Get all of the follow-up tests and care that your health care provider asks you to.

It may be helpful to bring this booklet with you. It discusses breast changes that are not cancer (**benign**), as well as changes that are abnormal or could be signs of cancer. Feel free to read different sections in this booklet as you need them. The "Words to know" section in the back of this booklet defines words that are shown in bold the first time they are used.

Words To Know

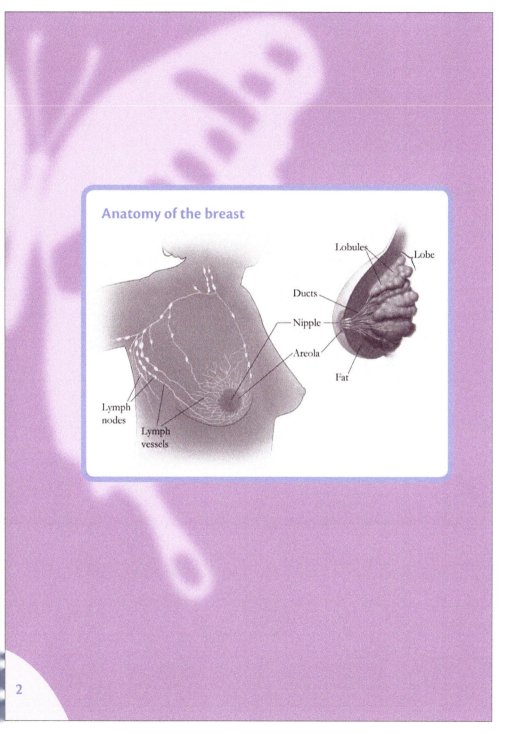

1 Breast and lymphatic system basics

To better understand breast changes, it helps to know what the breasts and **lymphatic system** are made of.

What are breasts made of?

Breasts are made of **connective tissue**, **glandular** tissue, and fatty tissue. Connective tissue and glandular tissue look dense, or white on a mammogram. Fatty tissue is non-dense, or black on a mammogram. **Dense breasts** can make mammograms harder to interpret.

Breasts have **lobes**, **lobules**, **ducts**, an areola, and a nipple.

- Lobes are sections of the glandular tissue. Lobes have smaller sections called lobules that end in tiny bulbs that can make milk.
- Ducts are thin tubes that connect the lobes and lobules. Milk flows from the lobules through the ducts to the nipple.
- The nipple is the small raised area at the tip of the breast. Milk flows through the nipple. The areola is the area of darker-colored skin around the nipple. Each breast also has **lymph vessels**.

What is the lymphatic system made of?

The lymphatic system, which is a part of your body's defense system, contains lymph vessels and lymph nodes.

- Lymph vessels are thin tubes that carry a fluid called **lymph** and **white blood cells**.
- Lymph vessels lead to small, bean-shaped organs called **lymph nodes**. Lymph nodes are found near your breast, under your arm, above your collarbone, in your chest, and in other parts of your body.
- Lymph nodes filter substances in lymph to help fight **infection** and disease. They also store disease-fighting white blood cells called **lymphocytes**.

Words To Know

2 Check with your health care provider about breast changes

Check with your health care provider if you notice that your breast looks or feels different. No change is too small to ask about. In fact, the best time to call is when you first notice a breast change.

Breast changes to see your health care provider about:

A lump (mass) or a firm feeling

- A lump in or near your breast or under your arm
- Thick or firm tissue in or near your breast or under your arm
- A change in the size or shape of your breast

Lumps come in different shapes and sizes. Most lumps are not cancer.

If you notice a lump in one breast, check your other breast. If both breasts feel the same, it may be normal. Normal breast tissue can sometimes feel lumpy.

Some women do regular **breast self-exams**. Doing breast self-exams can help you learn how your breasts normally feel and make it easier to notice and find any changes. Breast self-exams are not a substitute for mammograms.

Always get a lump checked. Don't wait until your next mammogram. You may need to have tests to be sure that the lump is not cancer.

4

Nipple discharge or changes

- Nipple discharge (fluid that is not breast milk)
- Nipple changes, such as a nipple that points or faces inward (inverted) into the breast

Nipple discharge may be different colors or textures. Nipple discharge is not usually a sign of cancer. It can be caused by birth control pills, some medicines, and infections.

Get nipple discharge checked, especially fluid that comes out by itself or fluid that is bloody.

Skin changes

- Itching, redness, scaling, dimples, or puckers on your breast

If the skin on your breast changes, get it checked as soon as possible.

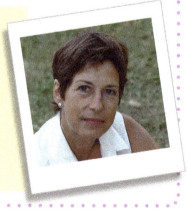

"I was in the shower one morning, when I felt a small lump in my breast. I was afraid and busy, but I didn't let that stop me. I made an appointment to see my doctor. I got the answers I needed."

Talk with your health care provider.

It can help to prepare before you meet with your health care provider.
Use the list below. Write down the breast changes you notice, as well as your **personal medical history** and your **family medical history** before your visit.

Tell your health care provider about breast changes or problems:

- These are the breast changes or problems I have noticed: _____
- This is what the breast change looks or feels like: _____
  (For example: Is the lump hard or soft? Does your breast feel tender or swollen? How big is the lump? What color is the nipple discharge?)
- This is where the breast change is: _____
  (For example: What part of the breast feels different? Do both breasts feel different or only one breast?)
- This is when I first noticed the breast change: _____
- Since then, this is the change I've noticed: _____
  (For example: Has it stayed the same or gotten worse?)

Share your personal medical history:

- I've had these breast problems in the past: _____
- These are the breast exams and tests that I have had: _____
- My last mammogram was on this date: _____
- My last menstrual period began on this date: _____
- These are the medicines or herbs that I take: _____
- Right now, I: ☐ Have breast implants   ☐ Am pregnant   ☐ Am breastfeeding
- I've had this type of cancer before: _____

Share your family medical history:

- My family members have had these breast problems or diseases: _____
- These family members had **breast cancer**: _____
- They were this old when they had breast cancer: _____

3 Breast changes during your lifetime that are not cancer

Most women have changes in their breasts during their lifetime. Many of these changes are caused by **hormones**. For example, your breasts may feel more lumpy or tender at different times in your **menstrual cycle**.

Other breast changes can be caused by the normal aging process. As you near **menopause**, your breasts may lose tissue and fat. They may become smaller and feel lumpy. Most of these changes are not cancer; they are called benign changes. However, if you notice a breast change, don't wait until your next mammogram. Make an appointment to get it checked.

Young women who have not gone through menopause often have more dense tissue in their breasts. Dense tissue has more glandular and connective tissue and less fat tissue. This kind of tissue makes mammograms harder to interpret—because both dense tissue and tumors show up as solid white areas on **x-ray** images. Breast tissue gets less dense as women get older.

Before or during your **menstrual periods**, your breasts may feel swollen, tender, or painful. You may also feel one or more lumps during this time because of extra fluid in your breasts. These changes usually go away by the end of your menstrual cycle. Because some lumps are caused by normal hormone changes, your health care provider may have you come back for a return visit, at a different time in your menstrual cycle.

During pregnancy, your breasts may feel lumpy. This is usually because the glands that produce milk are increasing in number and getting larger.

While breastfeeding, you may get a condition called **mastitis.** This happens when a milk duct becomes blocked. Mastitis causes the breast to look red and feel lumpy, warm, and tender. It may be caused by an infection and it is often treated with **antibiotics.** Sometimes the duct may need to be drained. If the redness or mastitis does not go away with treatment, call your health care provider.

As you approach menopause, your menstrual periods may come less often. Your hormone levels also change. This can make your breasts feel tender, even when you are not having your menstrual period. Your breasts may also feel more lumpy than they did before.

If you are taking hormones (such as menopausal hormone therapy, birth control pills, or injections) your breasts may become more dense. This can make a mammogram harder to interpret. Be sure to let your health care provider know if you are taking hormones.

When you stop having menstrual periods (menopause), your hormone levels drop, and your breast tissue becomes less dense and more fatty. You may stop having any lumps, pain, or nipple discharge that you used to have. And because your breast tissue is less dense, mammograms may be easier to interpret.

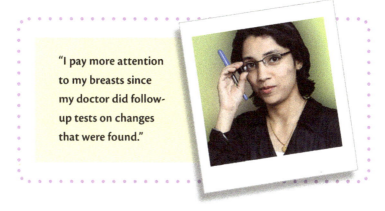

"I pay more attention to my breasts since my doctor did follow-up tests on changes that were found."

Finding breast changes

Here are some ways your health care provider can find breast changes:

Clinical breast exam

During a clinical breast exam, your health care provider checks your breasts and nipples and under your arms for any abnormal changes.

Ask your health care provider at what age and how often you should have a clinical breast exam. During the visit, it's important to share your personal medical history and your family medical history. This includes problems or diseases that you or family members have had.

Mammogram

A mammogram is an x-ray picture of your breast tissue. This test may find tumors that are too small to feel. During a mammogram, each breast is pressed between two plastic plates. Some discomfort is normal, but if it's painful, tell the **mammography** technician.

The best time to get a mammogram is at the end of your menstrual period. This is when your breasts are less tender. Some women have less breast tenderness if they don't have any caffeine for a couple of days before the mammogram.

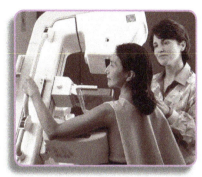

After the x-ray pictures are taken, they are sent to a **radiologist**, who studies them and sends a report to your health care provider.

Both film and digital mammography use x-rays to make a picture of the breast tissue. The actual procedure for getting the mammogram is the same. The difference is in how the images are recorded and stored. It's like the difference between a film camera and a digital camera.

- **Film mammography** stores the image directly on x-ray film.

- **Digital mammography** takes an electronic image of the breast and stores it directly in a computer. Digital images can be made lighter, darker, or larger. Images can also be stored and shared electronically.

A research study sponsored by the National Cancer Institute (NCI) showed that digital mammography and film mammography are about the same in terms of detecting breast cancer. However, digital mammography may be better at detecting breast cancer in women who are under age 50, have very dense breasts, or are **premenopausal** or **perimenopausal** (the times before and at the beginning of menopause).

Talk with your health care provider to learn more about what is best for you.

Mammograms are used for both screening and diagnosis.

◆ **Screening mammogram**

A **screening mammogram** is the kind of mammogram that most women get. It is used to find breast changes in women who have no signs of breast cancer.

◆ **Diagnostic mammogram**

If your recent screening mammogram found a breast change, or if a lump was found that needs to be checked, you may have a **diagnostic mammogram**. During a diagnostic mammogram, more x-ray pictures are taken to get views of the breast tissue from different angles. Certain areas of these pictures can also be made larger.

Mammograms and breast implants

When you make your appointment, be sure to tell the staff if you have **breast implants**. Ask if they have specialists who are trained in taking and reading mammograms of women with breast implants. This is important because breast implants can make it harder to see cancer or other abnormal changes on the mammogram. A special technique called **implant displacement views** is used.

◆ If you have breast implants for cosmetic reasons, you may have either a screening mammogram or a diagnostic mammogram. This will depend on the facility that does the mammogram.

◆ If you have breast implant(s) after having a **mastectomy** for breast cancer, talk with your breast **surgeon** or **oncologist** to learn about the best screening test for you.

Words To Know

MRI

Magnetic resonance imaging, also called **MRI**, uses a powerful magnet, radio waves, and a computer to take detailed pictures of areas inside the breast. MRI is another tool that can be used to find breast cancer. However, MRIs don't replace mammograms. They are used in addition to mammograms in women who are at increased risk of breast cancer.

MRIs have some limits. For example, they cannot find breast changes such as **microcalcifications**. MRIs are also less **specific** than other tests. This means that they may give **false-positive test results**—the test shows that there is cancer when there really is not.

Sometimes doctors recommend MRI for women who are at increased risk of breast cancer due to:

- Harmful changes (**mutations**) in the **BRCA1** or **BRCA2** gene
- A family history of breast cancer
- Your personal medical history

5 Getting your mammogram results

You should get a written report of your mammogram results within 30 days of your mammogram, since this is the law. Be sure the mammography facility has your address and phone number. It's helpful to get your mammogram at the same place each year. This way, your current mammogram can be compared with past mammograms.

If your results were normal:

- Your breast tissue shows no signs of a **mass** or **calcification**.
- Visit your health care provider if you notice a breast change before your next appointment.

If your results were abnormal:

- A breast change was found. It may be benign (not cancer), **premalignant** (may become cancer), or cancer.
- It's important to get all the follow-up tests your health care provider asks you to.

If you don't get your results, call your health care provider.

Keep in mind that most breast changes are not cancer. But all changes need to be checked, and more tests may be needed.

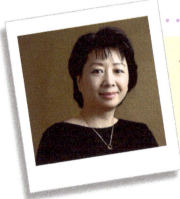

"I used to think when a mammogram found something, it was cancer. It turns out that most breast changes are *not* cancer."

What can a mammogram show?

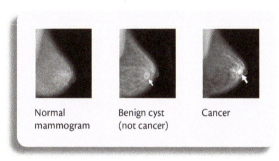

Normal mammogram | Benign cyst (not cancer) | Cancer

Mammograms can show lumps, **calcifications**, and other changes in your breast. The radiologist will study the mammogram for breast changes that do not look normal and for differences between your breasts. When possible, he or she will compare your most recent mammogram with past mammograms to check for changes.

Lump (or mass)

The size, shape, and edges of a lump give the radiologist important information. A lump that is not cancer often looks smooth and round and has a clear, defined edge. Lumps that look like this are often **cysts**. See the "Breast changes and conditions: Getting follow-up test results" section for more information about cysts. However, if the lump on the mammogram has a jagged outline and an irregular shape, more tests are needed.

Depending on the size and shape of the lump, your health care provider may ask you to have:

- Another clinical breast exam

- Another mammogram to have a closer look at the area

- An **ultrasound** exam to find out if the lump is solid or is filled with fluid

- A test called a **biopsy** to remove cells, or the entire lump, to look at under a **microscope** to check for signs of disease

14

Calcifications

Calcifications are deposits of **calcium** in the breast tissue. They are too small to be felt, but can be seen on a mammogram. There are two types:

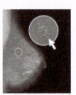

- **Macrocalcifications** look like small white dots on a mammogram. They are common in women over 50 years old. Macrocalcifications are not related to cancer and usually don't need more testing.

Calcium in your diet does not cause calcium deposits (calcifications) in the breast.

- **Microcalcifications** look like tiny white specks on a mammogram. They are usually not a sign of cancer. However, if they are found in an area of rapidly dividing cells, or grouped together in a certain way, you may need more tests.

Depending on how many calcifications you have, their size, and where they are found, your health care provider may ask you to have:

- Another mammogram to have a closer look at the area
- A test called a biopsy to check for signs of disease

Are mammogram results always right?

Mammography is a good tool to find breast changes in most women who have no signs of breast cancer. However, it does not detect all breast cancers, and many changes it finds are not cancer. See your health care provider if you have a lump that was not seen on a mammogram or notice any other breast changes.

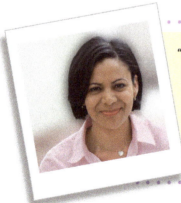

"Even though I was nervous, I'm glad I got the breast biopsy my doctor asked me to. As I waited for my results, it helped to remember the words of my doctor: 'Most breast changes are not cancer.'"

Words To Know

6 Follow-up tests to diagnose breast changes

An ultrasound exam, an MRI, a biopsy, or other follow-up tests may be needed to learn more about a breast change.

Ultrasound

An ultrasound exam uses sound waves to make a picture of breast tissue. This picture is called a **sonogram**. It helps radiologists to see if a lump or mass is solid or filled with fluid. A fluid-filled lump is called a cyst.

MRI

Magnetic resonance imaging, also called MRI, uses a powerful magnet, radio waves, and a computer to take detailed pictures of areas inside the breast. Sometimes breast lumps or large lymph nodes are found during a clinical breast exam or breast self-exam that were not seen on a mammogram or ultrasound. In these cases, an MRI can be used to learn more about these changes.

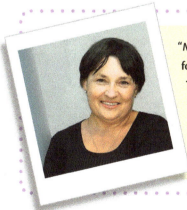

"My doctor said my mammogram found something 'abnormal.' That scared me, so I went back for more testing. It turned out that I had a benign cyst. It wasn't cancer. That was a relief."

Breast biopsy

A breast biopsy is a procedure to remove a sample of breast cells or tissue, or an entire lump. A **pathologist** then looks at the sample under a microscope to check for signs of disease. A biopsy is the only way to find out if cells are cancer.

Biopsies are usually done in an office or a clinic on an **outpatient** basis. This means you will go home the same day as the procedure. **Local anesthesia** is used for some biopsies. This means you will be awake, but you won't feel pain in your breast during the procedure. **General anesthesia** is often used for a **surgical biopsy**. This means that you will be asleep and won't wake up during the procedure.

Common types of breast biopsies:

◆ Fine-needle aspiration biopsy

A **fine-needle aspiration biopsy** is a simple procedure that takes only a few minutes. Your health care provider inserts a thin needle into the breast to take out fluid and cells.

◆ Core biopsy

A **core biopsy**, also called a core needle biopsy, uses a needle to remove small pieces or cores of breast tissue. The samples are about the size of a grain of rice. You may have a bruise, but usually not a scar.

◆ Vacuum-assisted biopsy

A **vacuum-assisted biopsy** uses a probe, connected to a vacuum device, to remove a small sample of breast tissue. The small cut made in the breast is much smaller than with surgical biopsy. This procedure causes very little scarring, and no stitches are needed.

Your doctor may use ultrasound or mammography during a breast biopsy to help locate the breast change.

Words To Know

◆ **Surgical biopsy**

A surgical biopsy is an operation to remove part, or all, of a lump so it can be looked at under a microscope to check for signs of disease. Sometimes a doctor will do a surgical biopsy as the first step. Other times, a doctor may do a surgical biopsy if the results of a needle biopsy do not give enough information.

When only a sample of breast tissue is removed, it's called an **incisional biopsy**. When the entire lump or suspicious area is removed, it's called an **excisional biopsy**.

If the breast change cannot be felt, **wire localization**, also called **needle localization,** may be used to find the breast change. During wire localization, a thin, hollow needle is inserted into the breast. A mammogram is taken to make sure that the needle is in the right place. Then a fine wire is inserted through the hollow needle, to mark the area of tissue to be removed. Next, the needle is removed, and another mammogram is taken. You then go to the operating room where the surgeon removes the wire and surrounding breast tissue. The tissue is sent to the lab to be checked for signs of disease.

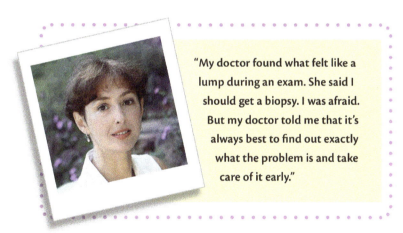

"My doctor found what felt like a lump during an exam. She said I should get a biopsy. I was afraid. But my doctor told me that it's always best to find out exactly what the problem is and take care of it early."

Questions to ask if a biopsy is recommended:

- Why is a biopsy needed? What will it tell us? _____
- What type of biopsy will I have? How will the biopsy be done? _____
- Where will the biopsy be done? How long will it take? _____
- Will it hurt? _____
- How much breast tissue will be removed? _____
- Will I be awake? _____
- What tests will be done on the breast tissue? _____
- When will I know the results? _____
- Will there be **side effects**? _____
- How should I care for the biopsy site? _____
- Will I need to rest after the biopsy? _____

Questions to ask about your biopsy results:

- What were the results of the biopsy? _____
- What do the biopsy results mean? _____
- What are the next steps? Do I need more tests? _____
- Who should I talk with next? _____
- Do I have an increased risk of breast cancer? _____
- Who can give me a second opinion on my biopsy results? _____

   Print out and take this list of questions with you when you talk with your health care provider.

Words To Know

7 Breast changes and conditions: Getting follow-up test results

Test results will tell if you have:

Breast changes that are not cancer

These changes are not cancer and do not increase your risk of breast cancer. They are called benign changes.

Adenosis: Small, round lumps, or a lumpy feeling that are caused by enlarged breast lobules. Sometimes the lumps are too small to be felt. If there is scar-like tissue, the condition may be painful and is called **sclerosing adenosis**.

Cysts: Lumps filled with fluid. Breast cysts often get bigger and may be painful just before your menstrual period begins. Cysts are most common in premenopausal women and in women who are taking menopausal hormone therapy.

Fat necrosis: Round, firm lumps that usually don't hurt. The lumps most often appear after an injury to the breast, surgery, or radiation therapy.

Fibroadenomas: Hard, round lumps that may feel like a small marble and move around easily. They are usually painless and are most common in young women under 30 years old.

Intraductal papilloma: A wart-like growth in a milk duct of the breast. It's usually found close to the nipple and may cause clear, sticky, or bloody discharge from the nipple. It may also cause pain and a lump. It is most common in women 35–55 years old.

Ask your doctor when you will get your test results. See the "Breast conditions and follow-up care" table to learn more about these conditions.

Breast changes that are <u>not</u> cancer, but increase your risk of cancer

These conditions are not cancer, but having them increases your risk of breast cancer. They are considered **risk factors** for breast cancer. Other risk factors include, for example, your age and a family history of breast cancer.

- **Atypical hyperplasia:**

    - **Atypical lobular hyperplasia (ALH)** is a condition in which abnormal cells are found in the breast lobules.

    - **Atypical ductal hyperplasia (ADH)** is a condition in which abnormal cells are found in the breast ducts.

- **Lobular carcinoma in situ (LCIS)** is a condition in which abnormal cells are found in the breast lobules. There are more abnormal cells in the lobule with LCIS than with ALH. Since these cells have not spread outside the breast lobules, it's called "**in situ**," which is a Latin term that means "in place."

The abnormal cells found in these conditions are not cancer cells. If you have ALH, ADH, or LCIS, talk with a doctor who specializes in breast health to make a plan that works best for you. Depending on your personal and family medical history, it may include:

- Mammograms every year

- Clinical breast exams every 6 to 12 months

- **Tamoxifen** (for all women) or **raloxifene** (for postmenopausal women). These drugs have been shown to lower some women's risk of breast cancer.

- Surgery. A small number of women with LCIS and high risk factors for breast cancer may choose to have surgery.

- **Clinical trials**. Talk with your health care provider about whether a clinical trial is a good choice for you.

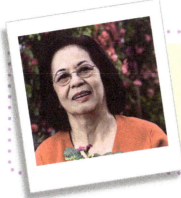

"Instead of stressing that something abnormal was found, I realized how lucky I was to have this small breast change found early."

Breast changes that may become cancer

Ductal carcinoma in situ (DCIS): DCIS is a condition in which abnormal cells are found in the lining of a breast duct. These cells have not spread outside the duct to the breast tissue. This is why it is called "in situ," which is a Latin term that means "in place." You may also hear DCIS called **Stage 0 breast carcinoma in situ** or **noninvasive** cancer.

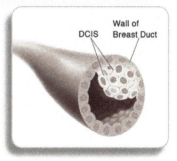

Since it's not possible to determine which cases of DCIS will become invasive breast cancer, it's important to get treatment for DCIS. Talk with a doctor who specializes in breast health to learn more. Treatment for DCIS is based on how much of the breast is affected, where DCIS is in the breast, and its **grade**. Most women with DCIS are cured with proper treatment.

Treatment choices for DCIS include:

♦ **Lumpectomy**. This is a type of **breast-conserving surgery** or **breast-sparing surgery**. It is usually followed by **radiation therapy**.

♦ **Mastectomy**. This type of surgery is used to remove the breast or as much of the breast tissue as possible.

♦ **Tamoxifen**. This drug may also be taken to lower the chance that DCIS will come back, or to prevent invasive breast cancer.

♦ Clinical trials. Talk with your health care provider about whether a clinical trial is a good choice for you.

I Don't Look Like What I've Been Through!

Breast cancer

Breast cancer is a disease in which cancer cells form in the tissues of the breast. Breast cancer cells:

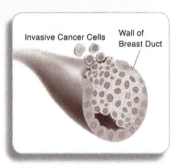

- Grow and divide without control
- Invade nearby breast tissue
- May form a mass called a **tumor**
- May **metastasize**, or spread, to the lymph nodes or other parts of the body

After breast cancer has been **diagnosed**, tests are done to find out the extent, or **stage**, of the cancer. The stage is based on the size of the tumor and whether the cancer has spread. Treatment depends on the stage of the cancer.

For more information about breast cancer and to get answers to any questions you may have, call **1-800-4-CANCER (1-800-422-6237)**. You can also go to NCI's **Breast Cancer Home Page** to learn more.

Get a second opinion

You may want to talk with another doctor to get a second opinion on your diagnosis or on your treatment. Many women do. And remember—it's important to talk with a doctor who specializes in breast cancer or in the breast condition that you have.

You can talk with your health care provider to find:

- Another pathologist to review your breast tissue slides and make a diagnosis
- Another surgeon, **radiation oncologist**, or **medical oncologist** to talk with about your treatment choices

Most doctors welcome a second opinion, especially when treatment is involved. Getting a second opinion is often covered, or even required, by your health insurance. Talking with another doctor can give you peace of mind. It can also help you make the best choices about your health.

23

8 Getting the support you need

It can be upsetting to notice a breast change, to get an abnormal test result, or to learn about a new condition or disease. We hope that the information in this booklet has answered some of your questions and calmed some of your fears as you talk with your health care provider and get the follow-up care you need.

Many women choose to get extra help and support for themselves. It may help to think about people who have been there for you during challenging times in the past.

- Ask friends or loved ones for support. Take someone with you while you are learning about your testing and treatment choices.

- Ask your health care provider to:
    - Explain medical terms that are new or confusing
    - Share with you how other people have handled the types of feelings that you are having
    - Tell you about specialists that you can talk with to learn more

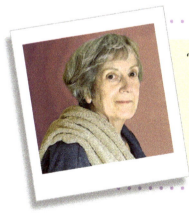

"I tried not to let the worries of tomorrow bother me today. It meant figuring out what I could and could not control. Talking with other women helped me."

Breast conditions and follow-up care

Condition	Features	What your doctor may recommend
Adenosis	• Small round lumps, lumpiness, or you may not feel anything at all • Enlarged breast lobules • If there is scar-like fibrous tissue, the condition is called sclerosing adenosis. It may be painful. • Some studies have found that women with sclerosing adenosis may have a slightly increased risk of breast cancer.	• A core biopsy or a surgical biopsy may be needed to make a diagnosis.
Atypical lobular hyperplasia (ALH)	• Abnormal cells in the breast lobules • ALH increases your risk of breast cancer.	Regular follow-up, such as: • Mammograms • Clinical breast exams Treatment, such as: • Tamoxifen (for all women) or raloxifene (for postmenopausal women)
Atypical ductal hyperplasia (ADH)	• Abnormal cells in the breast ducts • ADH increases your risk of breast cancer.	Regular follow-up, such as: • Mammograms • Clinical breast exams Treatment, such as: • Tamoxifen (for all women) or raloxifene (for postmenopausal women)

Words To Know

Breast conditions and follow-up care continued

Condition	Features	What your doctor may recommend
Breast cancer	• Cancer cells found in the breast, with a biopsy • A lump in or near your breast or under your arm • Thick or firm tissue in or near your breast or under your arm • A change in the size or shape of your breast • A nipple that's turned inward (inverted) into the breast • Skin on your breast that is itchy, red, scaly, dimpled, or puckered • Nipple discharge that is not breast milk	Treatment depends on the extent or stage of cancer. Tests are done to find out if the cancer has spread to others parts of your body. Treatment may include: • Surgery • **Chemotherapy** • Radiation therapy • **Hormonal therapy** • **Biological therapy** Clinical trials may be an option for you. Talk with your doctor to learn more.
Cysts	• Lumps filled with fluid • Often in both breasts • May be painful just before your menstrual period begins • Some cysts may be felt. Others are too small to be felt. • Most common in women 35–50 years old	• Cysts may be watched by your doctor over time, since they may go away on their own. • Ultrasound can show if the lump is solid or filled with fluid. • Fine needle aspiration may be used to remove fluid from the cyst.
Ductal carcinoma in situ (DCIS)	• Abnormal cells in the lining of a breast duct • Unlike cancer cells that can spread, these abnormal cells have not spread outside the breast duct. • May be called noninvasive cancer or Stage 0 breast carcinoma in situ.	Treatment is needed because doctors don't know which cases of DCIS may become invasive breast cancer. Treatment choices include: • Lumpectomy. This is a type of breast-conserving surgery or breast-sparing surgery. It is usually followed by radiation therapy. • Mastectomy. Surgery to remove the breast. • Tamoxifen. This drug may be taken to lower the chance that DCIS will come back after treatment or to prevent invasive breast cancer. • Clinical trials. Talk with your doctor about whether a clinical trial is a good choice for you.

Breast conditions and follow-up care continued

Condition	Features	What your doctor may recommend
Fat necrosis	• Round, firm lumps that usually don't hurt • May appear after an injury to the breast, surgery, or radiation therapy • Formed by damaged fatty tissue • Skin around the lump may look red, bruised, or dimpled • A benign (not cancer) breast condition	• A biopsy may be needed to diagnose and remove fat necrosis, since it often looks like cancer. • Fat necrosis does not usually need treatment.
Fibroadenoma	• Hard, round lumps that move around easily and usually don't hurt • Often found by the woman • Appear on a mammogram as smooth, round lumps with clearly defined edges • The most common benign breast tumors • Common in women under 30 years old • Most fibroadenomas do not increase your risk of breast cancer. However, complex fibroadenomas do slightly increase your risk.	• A biopsy may be needed to diagnose fibroadenoma. • A minimally invasive technique such as ultrasound-guided **cryoablation** or an excisional biopsy may be used to remove the lumps. • These growths may be watched by your doctor over time, since they may go away on their own.
Intraductal papilloma	• A wart-like growth inside the milk duct, usually close to the nipple • May cause pain and a lump • May cause clear, sticky, or bloody discharge • Most common in women 35–55 years old • Unlike single papillomas, multiple papillomas increase your risk of breast cancer.	• A biopsy may be needed to diagnose the growth and remove it.

Words To Know

Breast conditions and follow-up care continued

Condition	Features	What your doctor may recommend
Lobular carcinoma in situ (LCIS)	• A condition in which abnormal cells are found in the breast lobules • LCIS increases your risk of breast cancer.	Regular follow-up, such as: • Mammograms • Clinical breast exams Treatment choices: • Tamoxifen (for all women) or raloxifene (for postmenopausal women) may be taken. • A small number of women with LCIS and high risk factors for breast cancer may choose to have surgery. • Clinical trials may be an option for you. Talk with your doctor to learn more.
Macrocalcifications	• Calcium deposits in the breast that look like small white dots on a mammogram • Often caused by aging • Cannot be felt • Usually benign (not cancer) • Common in women over 50 years old	• Another mammogram may be needed to have a closer look at the area. • Treatment is usually not needed.
Microcalcifications	• Calcium deposits in the breast that look like tiny white specks on a mammogram • Not usually a sign of cancer. However, if found in an area of rapidly dividing cells or grouped together in a certain way, they may be a sign of DCIS or invasive breast cancer.	• Another mammogram or a biopsy may be needed to make a diagnosis.

I Don't Look Like What I've Been Through!

Resources to learn more

Find more organizations:
Visit NCI's database of National Organizations That Offer Cancer-Related Support Services to find organizations that provide emotional, practical, or financial support services to people with cancer and their families.

National Cancer Institute (NCI)

NCI has comprehensive research-based information on cancer prevention, screening, diagnosis, treatment, genetics, and supportive care. We also have a clinical trials database and can offer tailored searches.

Phone: 1-800-4-CANCER (1-800-422-6237)
Web site: **http://www.cancer.gov** or **http://www.cancer.gov/espanol**
Chat online: **livehelp.cancer.gov** (NCI's instant messaging service)
Email: **cancergovstaff@mail.nih.gov**

Order publications at **http://www.cancer.gov/publications** or by calling 1-800-4-CANCER

We invite you to call or go online to talk with our trained information specialists, who speak English or Spanish, to:

- Get answers to any cancer-related questions you may have
- Get free NCI publications
- Learn more about specific resources and organizations in your area
- Find information on the NCI Web site **http://www.cancer.gov**

American Cancer Society (ACS)

ACS gives cancer information and support to patients, families, and caregivers. It also supports research, community education, advocacy, and public policy issues. Trained cancer information specialists can answer questions about cancer, link you to resources in your community, and provide information on local events.

Phone: 1-800-ACS-2345 (1-800-227-2345)
TTY: 1-866-228-4327
Web site: **http://www.cancer.org**

Centers for Disease Control and Prevention (CDC)

CDC conducts, supports, and promotes efforts to prevent cancer and increase early detection of cancer. CDC's National Breast and Cervical Cancer Early Detection Program (NBCCEDP) provides these services for underserved women:

- Clinical breast exams
- Mammograms (free or low-cost)
- Diagnostic tests if results are abnormal
- Referrals to treatment

Toll Free: 1-800-CDC-INFO (1-800-232-4636)
TTY: 1-888-232-6348
Web site: **http://www.cdc.gov**

Words To Know

Centers for Medicare & Medicaid Services (CMS)

CMS provides information for consumers about patient rights, prescription drugs, and health insurance issues, including Medicare and Medicaid.

Medicare is health insurance for people age 65 or older, under age 65 with certain disabilities, and any age with permanent kidney failure. It covers an annual screening mammogram, among other services. Medicare has information about providers in your area. English- or Spanish-speaking representatives can help you.

Phone:	1-800-MEDICARE (1-800-633-4227)
TTY:	1-877-486-2048
Web site:	**http://www.cms.hhs.gov**

Medicaid is a program for people who need financial help with medical bills. You can learn more about this program by calling your local state welfare offices, state health department, state social services agencies, or your state's Medicaid office. Spanish-speaking staff is available in some offices.

Web site: **http://www.medicaid.gov**

National Women's Health Information Center (NWHIC)

NWHIC is a gateway to women's health information. NWHIC has English- and Spanish-speaking Information and Referral Specialists who will order free health information for you. They can also help you find organizations that can answer your health-related questions.

Phone:	1-800-994-9662
TDD:	1-888-220-5446
Web site:	**http://www.womenshealth.gov**

U.S. Food and Drug Administration (FDA)

The FDA has fact sheets and brochures about mammography, as well as information about a certified mammography facility near you. It also has laws about how these facilities are run.

Phone:	1-888-INFO-FDA (1-888-463-6332)
Web site:	**http://www.fda.gov**

Words To Know

abnormal: Not normal. An abnormal lesion or growth may be cancer, premalignant (may become cancer), or benign (not cancer).

adenosis: A disease or abnormal change in a gland. Breast adenosis is a benign condition in which the lobules are larger than usual.

ADH (atypical ductal hyperplasia): A benign (not cancer) condition in which there are more cells than normal in the lining of breast ducts and the cells look abnormal under a microscope. Having ADH increases your risk of breast cancer.

ALH (atypical lobular hyperplasia): A benign (not cancer) condition in which there are more cells than normal in the breast lobules and the cells look abnormal under a microscope. Having ALH increases your risk of breast cancer.

antibiotic: A drug used to treat infections caused by bacteria and other microorganisms.

areola: The area of dark-colored skin on the breast that surrounds the nipple.

atypical hyperplasia: A benign (not cancer) condition in which cells look abnormal under a microscope and are increased in number.

Words To Know

benign: Not cancer. Benign tumors may grow larger but do not spread to other parts of the body.

biological therapy: Treatment to boost or restore the ability of the immune system to fight cancer, infections, and other diseases. Also used to lessen certain side effects that may be caused by some cancer treatments. Agents used in biological therapy include monoclonal antibodies, growth factors, and vaccines. These agents may also have a direct antitumor effect. Also called biological response modifier therapy, biotherapy, BRM therapy, and immunotherapy.

biopsy: The removal of cells or tissues for examination by a pathologist. The pathologist may study the tissue under a microscope or perform other tests on the cells or tissue. There are many different types of biopsy procedures. The most common types include: (1) incisional biopsy, in which only a sample of tissue is removed; (2) excisional biopsy, in which an entire lump or suspicious area is removed; and (3) needle biopsy, in which a sample of tissue or fluid is removed with a needle. When a wide needle is used, the procedure is called a core biopsy. When a thin needle is used, the procedure is called a fine-needle aspiration biopsy.

BRCA1: A gene on chromosome 17 that normally helps to suppress cell growth. A person who inherits certain mutations (changes) in a BRCA1 gene has a higher risk of getting breast, ovarian, prostate, and other types of cancer. BRCA1 is short for (**br**east **ca**ncer **1**, early onset gene).

BRCA2: A gene on chromosome 13 that normally helps to suppress cell growth. A person who inherits certain mutations (changes) in a BRCA2 gene has a higher risk of getting breast, ovarian, prostate, and other types of cancer. BRCA2 is short for (**br**east **ca**ncer **2**, early onset gene).

breast: Glandular organ located on the chest. The breast is made up of connective tissue, fat, and glandular tissue that can make milk. Also called mammary gland.

breast cancer: Cancer that forms in tissues of the breast, usually the ducts (tubes that carry milk to the nipple) and lobules (glands that make milk). It occurs in both men and women, although male breast cancer is rare.

breast density: Describes the relative amount of different tissues present in the breast. A dense breast has less fat than glandular and connective tissue. Mammogram films of breasts with higher density are harder to read and interpret than those of less dense breasts.

breast duct: A thin tube in the breast that carries milk from the breast lobules to the nipple. Also called milk duct.

breast implant: A silicone gel-filled or saline-filled sac placed under the chest muscle to restore breast shape.

breast-conserving surgery: An operation to remove the breast cancer but not the breast itself. Types of breast-conserving surgery include lumpectomy (removal of the lump), quadrantectomy (removal of one quarter, or quadrant, of the breast), and segmental mastectomy (removal of the cancer as well as some of the breast tissue around the tumor and the lining over the chest muscles below the tumor). Also called breast-sparing surgery.

breast self-exam: An exam by a woman of her breasts to check for lumps or other changes. Also called BSE.

breast-sparing surgery: An operation to remove the breast cancer but not the breast itself. Types of breast-sparing surgery include lumpectomy (removal of the lump), quadrantectomy (removal of one quarter, or quadrant, of the breast), and segmental mastectomy (removal of the cancer as well as some of the breast tissue around the tumor and the lining over the chest muscles below the tumor). Also called breast-conserving surgery.

calcification: Deposits of calcium in the tissues. Calcification in the breast can be seen on a mammogram but cannot be felt. There are two types of breast calcifications, macrocalcification and microcalcification. Macrocalcifications are large deposits of calcium and are usually not related to cancer. Microcalcifications are specks of calcium that may be found in an area of rapidly dividing cells. Many microcalcifications clustered together may be a sign of cancer.

calcium: A mineral needed for healthy teeth, bones, and other body tissues. It is the most common mineral in the body. A deposit of calcium in body tissues, such as breast tissue, may be a sign of disease.

cancer: A term for diseases in which abnormal cells divide without control and can invade nearby tissues. Cancer cells can also spread to other parts of the body through the blood and lymph systems.

chemotherapy: Treatment with drugs that kill cancer cells.

clinical breast exam: A physical exam of the breast performed by a health care provider to check for lumps or other changes. Also called CBE.

clinical trial: A type of research study that tests how well new medical approaches work in people. A clinical trial tests new method of screening, prevention, diagnosis, or treatment of a disease. Also called clinical study.

core biopsy: The removal of a tissue sample with a wide needle for examination under a microscope. Also called core needle biopsy.

connective tissue: Supporting tissue that surrounds other tissues and organs. Specialized connective tissue includes bone, cartilage, blood, and fat

cryoablation: A procedure in which tissue is frozen to destroy abnormal cells. This is usually done with a special instrument that contains liquid nitrogen or liquid carbon dioxide. Also called cryosurgery.

cyst: A sac or capsule in the body. It may be filled with fluid or other material.

DCIS (ductal carcinoma in situ): A noninvasive condition in which abnormal cells are found in the lining of a breast duct. The abnormal cells have not spread outside the duct to other tissues in the breast. In some cases, DCIS may become invasive cancer and spread to other tissues, although it is not known at this time how to predict which lesions will become invasive. Also called intraductal carcinoma.

dense breasts: See breast density.

diagnosis: The process of identifying a disease, such as cancer, from its signs and symptoms.

diagnostic mammogram: X-ray of the breasts used to check for cancer after a lump or other sign or symptom of breast cancer has been found.

digital mammography: A technique that uses a computer, rather than x-ray film, to record x-ray images of the breast.

duct: See breast duct.

excisional biopsy: A surgical procedure in which an entire lump or suspicious area is removed for diagnosis. The tissue is then examined under a microscope to check for signs of disease.

false-positive test result: A test result that indicates that a person has a specific disease or condition when the person actually does not have the disease or condition.

family medical history: A record of the relationships among family members along with their medical histories. This includes current and past illnesses. A family medical history may show a pattern of certain diseases in a family. Also called family history.

fat necrosis: A benign condition in which fat tissue in the breast or other organs is damaged by injury, surgery, or radiation therapy. The fat tissue in the breast may be replaced by a cyst or by scar tissue, which may feel like a round, firm lump. The skin around the lump may look red, bruised, or dimpled.

fibroadenoma: A benign (not cancer) tumor that usually forms in the breast from both fibrous and glandular tissue. Fibroadenomas are the most common benign breast tumors.

film mammography: The use of x-rays to create a picture of the breast on a film.

fine-needle aspiration biopsy: The removal of tissue or fluid with a thin needle for examination under a microscope. Also called FNA biopsy.

general anesthesia: A temporary loss of feeling and a complete loss of awareness that feels like a very deep sleep. It is caused by special drugs or other substances called anesthetics. General anesthesia stops patients from feeling pain during surgery or other procedures.

gland: An organ that makes one or more substances, such as milk, hormones, digestive juices, sweat, tears, or saliva.

glandular: See gland.

grade: A description of a tumor based on how abnormal the cancer cells look under a microscope and how quickly the tumor is likely to grow and spread. Grading systems are different for each type of cancer.

hormonal therapy: Treatment that adds, blocks, or removes hormones. For certain conditions (such as diabetes or menopause), hormones are given to adjust low hormone levels. To slow or stop the growth of certain cancers (such as prostate and breast cancer), synthetic hormones or other drugs may be given to block the body's natural hormones. Sometimes surgery is needed to remove the gland that makes a certain hormone. Also called endocrine therapy, hormone therapy, and hormone treatment.

hormone: One of many chemicals made by glands in the body. Hormones circulate in the bloodstream and control the actions of certain cells or organs. Some hormones can also be made in the laboratory.

implant displacement views: A procedure used to do a mammogram (x-ray of the breasts) in women with breast implants. The implant is pushed back against the chest wall and the breast tissue is pulled forward and around it so the tissue can be seen in the mammogram. Also called Eklund displacement views and Eklund views.

in situ: In its original place. For example, in carcinoma in situ, abnormal cells are found only in the place where they first formed. They have not spread.

incisional biopsy: A surgical procedure in which a portion of a lump or suspicious area is removed for diagnosis. The tissue is then examined under a microscope to check for signs of disease.

infection: Invasion and multiplication of germs in the body. Infections can occur in any part of the body and can spread throughout the body. The germs may be bacteria, viruses, yeast, or fungi. They can cause a fever and other problems, depending on where the infection occurs.

When the body's natural defense system is strong, it can often fight the germs and prevent infection. Some cancer treatments can weaken the natural defense system.

intraductal papilloma: A benign (not cancer), wart-like growth in a milk duct of the breast. It is usually found close to the nipple and may cause a discharge from the nipple. It may also cause

pain and a lump in the breast that can be felt. It usually affects women aged 35-55 years. Having a single papilloma does not increase the risk of breast cancer. When there are multiple intraductal breast papillomas, they are usually found farther from the nipple. There may not be a nipple discharge and the papillomas may not be felt. Having multiple intraductal breast papillomas may increase the risk of breast cancer. Also called intraductal breast papilloma.

LCIS (lobular carcinoma in situ): A condition in which abnormal cells are found in the lobules of the breast. LCIS seldom becomes invasive cancer; however, having it in one breast increases the risk of developing breast cancer in either breast.

lobe: A portion of an organ, such as the breast, liver, lung, thyroid, or brain.

lobule: A small lobe or a subdivision of a lobe.

local anesthesia: A temporary loss of feeling in one small area of the body caused by special drugs or other substances called anesthetics. The patient stays awake but has no feeling in the area of the body treated with the anesthetic.

lumpectomy: Surgery to remove abnormal tissue or cancer from the breast and a small amount of normal tissue around it. It is a type of breast-sparing surgery.

lymph: The clear fluid that travels through the lymphatic system and carries cells that help fight infections and other diseases. Also called lymphatic fluid.

lymph node: A rounded mass of lymphatic tissue that is surrounded by a capsule of connective tissue. Lymph nodes filter lymph (lymphatic fluid), and they store lymphocytes (white blood cells). They are located along lymph vessels. Also called a lymph gland.

lymph vessel: A thin tube that carries lymph (lymphatic fluid) and white blood cells through the lymphatic system. Also called lymphatic vessel.

lymphatic system: The tissues and organs that produce, store, and carry white blood cells that fight infections and other diseases. This system includes the bone marrow, spleen, thymus, lymph nodes, and lymph vessels (a network of thin tubes that carry lymph and white blood cells). Lymph vessels branch, like blood vessels, into all the tissues of the body.

lymphocyte: A type of immune cell that is made in the bone marrow and is found in the blood and in lymph tissue. The two main types of lymphocytes are B lymphocytes and T lymphocytes. B lymphocytes make antibodies, and T lymphocytes help kill tumor cells and help control immune responses. A lymphocyte is a type of white blood cell.

macrocalcification: A small deposit of calcium in the breast that cannot be felt but can be seen on a mammogram. It is usually caused by aging, an old injury, or inflamed tissue and is usually not related to cancer.

mammogram: An x-ray of the breast.

mammography: The use of x-rays to create a picture of the breast tissue.

mass: In medicine, a lump in the body. It may be caused by the abnormal growth of cells, a cyst, hormonal changes, or an immune reaction. A mass may be benign (not cancer) or malignant (cancer).

mastectomy: Surgery to remove the breast, or as much of the breast tissue as possible.

mastitis: A condition in which breast tissue is inflamed. It is usually caused by an infection and is most often seen in nursing mothers.

medical oncologist: A doctor who specializes in diagnosing and treating cancer using chemotherapy, hormonal therapy, and biological therapy. A medical oncologist often is the main health care provider for someone who has cancer. A medical oncologist also gives supportive care and may coordinate treatment given by other specialists.

menopause: The time of life when a woman's ovaries stop working and menstrual periods stop. Natural menopause usually occurs around age 50. A woman is said to be in menopause when she hasn't had a period for 12 months in

Words To Know

a row. Symptoms of menopause include hot flashes, mood swings, night sweats, vaginal dryness, trouble concentrating, and infertility.

menopausal hormone therapy: Hormones (estrogen, progesterone, or both) given to women after menopause to replace the hormones no longer produced by the ovaries. Also called hormone replacement therapy and HRT.

menstrual cycle: The monthly cycle of hormonal changes from the beginning of one menstrual period to the beginning of the next.

menstrual period: The periodic discharge of blood and tissue from the uterus. From puberty until menopause, menstruation occurs about every 28 days, but does not occur during pregnancy.

metastasize: To spread from one part of the body to another. When cancer cells metastasize and form secondary tumors, the cells in the metastatic tumor are like those in the original (primary) tumor.

microcalcification: A tiny deposit of calcium in the breast that cannot be felt but can be detected on a mammogram. A cluster of these very small specks of calcium may indicate that cancer is present.

microscope: An instrument that is used to look at cells and other small objects that cannot be seen with the eye alone.

MRI (magnetic resonance imaging): A procedure in which radio waves and a powerful magnet linked to a computer are used to create detailed pictures of areas inside the body. These pictures can show the difference between normal and diseased tissue. MRI makes better images of organs and soft tissue than other scanning techniques, such as computed tomography (CT) or x-ray. MRI is especially useful for imaging the brain, the spine, the soft tissue of joints, and the inside of bones. Also called NMRI and nuclear magnetic resonance imaging.

mutation: Any change in the DNA of a cell. Mutations may be caused by mistakes during cell division, or they may be caused by exposure to DNA-damaging agents in the environment. Mutations can be harmful, beneficial, or have no effect. If they occur in cells that make eggs or sperm, they can be inherited; if mutations occur in other types of cells, they are not inherited. Certain mutations may lead to cancer or other diseases.

needle localization: A procedure used to mark a small area of abnormal tissue so it can be removed by surgery. An imaging device is used to guide a thin wire with a hook at the end through a hollow needle to place the wire in or around the abnormal area. Once the wire is in the right place, the needle is removed and the wire is left in place so the doctor will know where the abnormal tissue is. The wire is removed at the time the biopsy is done. Also called needle/wire localization and wire localization.

nipple: In anatomy, the small raised area in the center of the breast through which milk can flow to the outside.

nipple discharge: Fluid coming from the nipple that is not breast milk.

noninvasive: In cancer, it describes disease that has not spread outside the tissue in which it began. In medicine, it describes a procedure that does not require inserting an instrument through the skin or into a body opening.

oncologist: A doctor who specializes in treating cancer. Some oncologists specialize in a particular type of cancer treatment. For example, a radiation oncologist specializes in treating cancer with radiation.

outpatient: A patient who visits a health care facility for diagnosis or treatment without spending the night. Sometimes called a day outpatient.

pathologist: A doctor who identifies diseases by studying cells and tissues under a microscope.

perimenopausal: Describes the time in a woman's life when menstrual periods become irregular as she approaches menopause. This is usually three to five years before menopause and is often marked by many of the symptoms of menopause, including hot flashes, mood swings, night sweats, vaginal dryness, trouble concentrating, and infertility.

personal medical history: A collection of information about a person's health. It may include information about allergies, illnesses and surgeries, and dates and results of physical exams, tests, screenings, and immunizations. It may also include information about medicines taken and about diet and exercise. Also called personal health record and personal history.

premalignant: A term used to describe a condition that may (or is likely to) become cancer. Also called precancerous.

premenopausal: Having to do with the time before menopause. Menopause ("change of life") is the time of life when a woman's menstrual periods stop permanently.

radiation oncologist: A doctor who specializes in using radiation to treat cancer.

radiation therapy: The use of high-energy radiation from x-rays, gamma rays, neutrons, protons, and other sources to destroy cancer cells and shrink tumors. Radiation may come from a machine outside the body (external-beam radiation therapy), or it may come from radioactive material placed in the body near cancer cells (internal radiation therapy).

radiologist: A doctor who specializes in creating and interpreting pictures of areas inside the body. The pictures are produced with x-rays, sound waves, or other types of energy.

raloxifene: The active ingredient in a drug used to reduce the risk of invasive breast cancer in postmenopausal women who are at high risk of the disease or who have osteoporosis. It is also used to prevent and treat osteoporosis in postmenopausal women. It is also being studied in the prevention of breast cancer in certain premenopausal women and in the prevention and treatment of other conditions. Raloxifene blocks the effects of the hormone estrogen in the breast and increases the amount of calcium in bone. It is a type of selective estrogen receptor modulator (SERM).

risk factor: Something that may increase the chance of developing a disease. Some examples of risk factors for cancer include age, a family history of certain cancers, use of tobacco products, certain eating habits, obesity, lack of exercise, exposure to radiation or other cancer-causing agents, and certain genetic changes.

sclerosing adenosis: A benign condition in which scar-like tissue is found in a gland, such as the breast lobules or the prostate. A biopsy may be needed to tell the difference between the abnormal tissue and cancer. Women with sclerosing adenosis of the breast may have a slightly increased risk of breast cancer.

screening: Checking for disease when there are no symptoms. Since screening may find diseases at an early stage, there may be a better chance of curing the disease. Examples of cancer screening tests are the mammogram (breast), colonoscopy (colon), Pap smear (cervix), and PSA blood level and digital rectal exam (prostate). Screening can also include checking for a person's risk of developing an inherited disease by doing a genetic test.

screening mammogram: X-rays of the breasts taken to check for breast cancer in the absence of signs or symptoms.

side effect: A problem that occurs when treatment affects healthy tissues or organs. Some common side effects of cancer treatment are fatigue, pain, nausea, vomiting, decreased blood cell counts, hair loss, and mouth sores.

sonogram: A computer picture of areas inside the body created by bouncing high-energy sound waves (ultrasound) off internal tissues or organs. Also called an ultrasonogram.

specific: See specificity.

specificity: When referring to a medical test, specificity refers to the percentage of people who test negative for a specific disease among a group of people who do not have the disease. No test is 100% specific because some people who do not have the disease will test positive for it (false positive).

stage: The extent of a cancer in the body. Staging is usually based on the size of the tumor, whether lymph nodes contain cancer, and whether the cancer has spread from the original site to other parts of the body.

stage 0 breast carcinoma in situ: There are 2 types of stage 0 breast cancer: ductal carcinoma in situ (DCIS) and lobular carcinoma in situ (LCIS). DCIS is a noninvasive condition in which abnormal cells are found in the lining of a breast duct (a tube that carries milk to the nipple). The abnormal cells have not spread outside the duct to other tissues in the breast. In some cases, DCIS may spread to other tissues, although it is not known how to predict which lesions will become invasive cancer. LCIS is a condition in which abnormal cells are found in the lobules (small sections of tissue involved with making milk) of the breast. This condition seldom becomes invasive cancer; however, having LCIS in one breast increases the risk of developing breast cancer in either breast. Stage 0 breast cancer is also called breast carcinoma in situ.

surgeon: A doctor who removes or repairs a part of the body by operating on the patient.

surgery: A procedure to remove or repair a part of the body or to find out whether disease is present. Also called an operation.

surgical biopsy: The removal of tissue by a surgeon for examination by a pathologist. The pathologist may study the tissue under a microscope.

tamoxifen: A drug used to treat certain types of breast cancer in women and men. It is also used to prevent breast cancer in women who have had (DCIS) ductal carcinoma in situ (abnormal cells in the ducts of the breast) and women who are high risk of developing breast cancer. Tamoxifen is also being studied in the treatment of other types of cancer. It blocks the effects of the hormone estrogen in the breast. Tamoxifen is a type of antiestrogen. Also called tamoxifen citrate.

tumor: An abnormal mass of tissue that results when cells divide more than they should or do not die when they should. Tumors may be benign (not cancer), or malignant (cancer). Also called neoplasm.

ultrasound: A procedure in which high-energy sound waves are bounced off internal tissues or organs and make echoes. The echo patterns are shown on the screen of an ultrasound machine, forming a picture of body tissues called a sonogram. Also called an ultrasonography.

vacuum-assisted biopsy: A procedure in which a small sample of tissue is removed from the breast. An imaging device is used to guide a hollow probe connected to a vacuum device. The probe is inserted through a tiny cut made in numbed skin on the breast. The tissue sample is removed using gentle vacuum suction and a small rotating knife within the probe. Then the tissue sample is studied under a microscope to check for signs of disease. This procedure causes very little scarring and no stitches are needed. Also called VACB and vacuum-assisted core biopsy.

white blood cell: A type of immune cell. Most white blood cells are made in the bone marrow and are found in the blood and lymph tissue. White blood cells help the body fight infections and other diseases. Granulocytes, monocytes, and lymphocytes are white blood cells. Also called leukocyte and WBC.

wire localization: A procedure used to mark a small area of abnormal tissue so it can be removed by surgery. An imaging device is used to guide a thin wire with a hook at the end through a hollow needle to place the wire in or around the abnormal area. Once the wire is in the right place, the needle is removed and the wire is left in place so the doctor will know where the abnormal tissue is. The wire is removed when a biopsy is done. Also called needle localization and needle/wire localization.

x-ray: A type of high-energy radiation. In low doses, x-rays are used to diagnose diseases by making pictures of the inside of the body. In high doses, x-rays are used to treat cancer.

Bibliography

Action. (n.d.) In *Merriam-Webster's collegiate dictionary*. Retrieved from http://www.merriam-webster.com/dictionary/Action

Albert Einstein. (n.d.) Wisdom Quotes. Retrieved from http://wisdomquotes.com/alberteinstein

Benjamin E. Mays Quotes. (n.d.). BrainyQuote.com. Retrieved April 27, 2018, from BrainyQuote.com Web site: https://www.brainyquote.com/quotes/benjamin_e_mays_610662

Complacency. (n.d.) In *Merriam-Webster's collegiate dictionary*. Retrieved from http://www.merriam-webster.com/dictionary/Complacency

Excuse. (n.d.) In *Merriam-Webster's collegiate dictionary*. Retrieved from http://www.merriam-webster.com/dictionary/Excuse

The Holy **Bible**, King James Version. Chicago: Moody Publishers, 1994

Iyanla Vanzant Quotes. (n.d.). BrainyQuote.com. Retrieved November 27, 2017, from Brainy Quote. Web site: https://www.brainyquote.com/quotes/iyanla_vanzant_519985

Mahatma Gandhi. (n.d.) www.goodreads.com/quotes/mahatmagandhi

New Living Version. Bible Gateway, www.biblegateway.com. Accessed 30 June. 2017.

Peterson, Eugene H. *The Message.* Bible Gateway, www.biblegateway.com. Accessed 19 Jul. 2018.

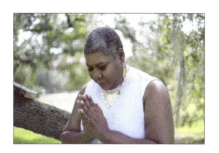

About the Author

Deborah Thomas is a mother of three and a grandmother. She's a professor at Strayer University and works as a supervisor in the transportation industry. She is a praying woman who is devoted to the Word of God and is persistent about sharing what God has done in her life and passes that hope to others. Her passion is teaching, and she loves to share the Word of God. She's a college graduate with a bachelor's degree in business and a Master of Divinity from Asbury Seminary. She resides in Orlando, Florida. If you don't catch her doing the things mentioned above, she enjoys sports, reading, and hanging out with Autumn, her granddaughter.

CPSIA information can be obtained
at www.ICGtesting.com
Printed in the USA
JSHW021524080120
3438JS00001B/2

9 781545 662922